GOLF PERFORMANCE TRAINING

GOLF PERFORMANCE TRAINING

... What They Won't Tell You

GARY BANNISTER, M.ED.

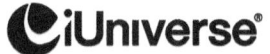

GOLF PERFORMANCE TRAINING
… WHAT THEY WON'T TELL YOU

iUniverse books may be ordered through booksellers or by contacting:

iUniverse
1663 Liberty Drive
Bloomington, IN 47403
www.iuniverse.com
1-800-Authors (1-800-288-4677)

Because of the dynamic nature of the Internet, any web addresses or links contained in this book may have changed since publication and may no longer be valid. The views expressed in this work are solely those of the author and do not necessarily reflect the views of the publisher, and the publisher hereby disclaims any responsibility for them.

Any people depicted in stock imagery provided by Thinkstock are models, and such images are being used for illustrative purposes only.
Certain stock imagery © Thinkstock.

ISBN: 978-1-4917-8941-4 (sc)
ISBN: 978-1-4917-8942-1 (hc)
ISBN: 978-1-4917-8940-7 (e)

Library of Congress Control Number: 2016903628

Print information available on the last page.

iUniverse rev. date: 04/14/2016

To my mother, Beverly Bannister, who recently passed at the age of ninety-two. A beautiful woman and loving mom, she provided her family with everything – education, love and support.

A single regret: She never revealed the secret to her putting prowess.

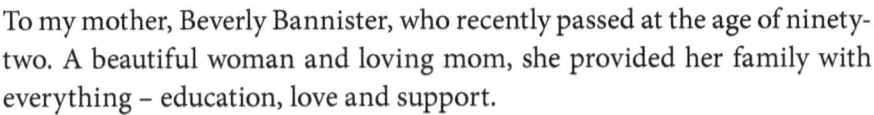

To my best friend and partner, Judy Barre, who recently passed, victim of a stroke. Beautiful, caring, friendly and kind, she focused her limitless energy on the well-being of others and exceeded my expectations every day for twenty-one years. Truly one-of-a-kind and a joy to be around, she leaves behind a loving family and wonderful memories.

CONTENTS

List of Illustrations... ix

List of Tables x

Acknowledgements... xi

Introduction...xiii

Front Nine (Out)

Hole #1: Improving Functional Ability in Golf............................3
Hole #2: Skill Acquisition.. 10
Hole #3: The Potential Benefits of Exercise 23
Hole #4: A Strategy 35
Hole #5: Strength Training Principles................................. 44
Hole #6: Skill Training vs Strength Training.......................... 51
Hole #7: Functional Training 56
Hole #8: Functional Training for Golf 68
Hole #9: Functional Training vs Traditional Training.............. 90

Back Nine (In)

Hole #10: Core Training 103
Hole #11: The Low-Back Hoax..117
Hole #12: Full-Range Exercise 132
Hole #13: *Real* Functional Training....................................141
Hole #14: Proper Strength Training for Golf...........................148
Hole #15: Advanced Training for Golf 166
Hole #16: Avoiding Hazards... 182
Hole #17: The Home Stretch 195
Hole #18: From The Neck Up 205

A Wee Nip

The 19th Hole: Home at Last 219

Notes 227

Bibliography..229

Index 235

LIST OF ILLUSTRATIONS

Front Nine (Out)

Hole #8:

      Figure 1: Slow Speed of Movement 79

      Figure 2: Fast Speed of Movement..79

Back Nine (In)

Hole #11:

      Figure 1: Muscle Isolation - Pelvic Restraint 120

Hole #17: Stretches

      Figure 1: Overhead Reach.. 198

      Figure 2: Side-Bend.. 198

      Figure 3: Behind-Head Reach...199

      Figure 4: Trunk Rotation 199

      Figure 5: Calf Stretch 201

      Figure 6: Soleus Stretch 201

      Figure 7: Standing Hamstring Stretch 202

      Figure 8: Deep Squat..202

      Figure 9: Seated Groin Stretch 203

      Figure 10: Seated Hamstring Stretch 203

      Figure 11: Forearm Stretch 204

A Wee Nip

LIST OF TABLES

Front Nine (Out)

Hole #4:

Figure 1: Effect of Supplemental Exercise on Trainable
Performance Factors 42

Hole #9:

Figure 1: Functional Exercise versus Traditional Exercise 98

Back Nine (In)

Hole #11:

Figure 2: Risk Factors For Spinal Injury 121
Figure 3: Lumbar Extension (MedX) 122
Figure 4: Lumbar Extension (Nautilus) 123
Figure 5: The Effect Of Training With Pelvic
Stabilization On Lumbar Extension Strength 124
Figure 6: Strength Gains (Lumbar Extension)..........................126
Figure 7: Strength Maintenance (Lumbar Extension) 127

Hole #12:

Figure 1: Barbell versus Nautilus® Curl 135
Figure 2: Requirements for Full-Range Exercise 139

Hole #14:

Figure 1: Prime Movers.. 149
Figure 2: Strength Training Principles...................................... 153

Hole #15:

Figure 1: Reaching Strength Potential....................................... 180

A Wee Nip

Hole #19:

Figure 1: Scorecard 225

ACKNOWLEDGEMENTS

C PGA professional, Gordon McInnis, Sr. introduced me to the Royal and Ancient game when I was fourteen. Inducted into the Ontario Golf Hall of Fame in 2001 for his work with Marlene Stewart Streit and Cathy Sherk, *Senior* was head professional at Lookout Point Golf and Country Club in Fonthill, Ontario for fifty-four years. He provided a simple foundation for many with his focus on balance, rhythm and *The Swing's the Thing*. A special man dedicated to his craft.

My brother, Alan Bannister - older by a year and a half - inspired me with his athletic talent, especially his ability to play golf, then and now. His humor, friendship and love of family have, so often, come to the rescue.

My thesis advisor, Celeste Ulrich, Ph.D., University of North Carolina at Greensboro, identified and encouraged my talent for writing, and went beyond the call of duty to secure my first teaching position.

Digby Sale, Ph.D., my exercise physiology professor at McMaster University in Hamilton, Ontario, cultivated an interest in his subject, and first introduced me to a Nautilus® machine.

McMaster University golf coach, John Carruthers, loved the challenge of the game and motivated his team to perform. Often my partner in matches, he provided plenty of encouragement - a great athlete and competitor.

Michael N. Fulton, M.D., orthopedic representative for Nautilus Sports/ Medical Industries and MedX Corporation, assisted and inspired many by his unwavering belief in the value of progressive resistance exercise. I cherish his expertise and friendship.

Edward B. Homsey, archivist of the Walter J. Travis Society, for allowing use of the picture of Walter J. Travis on the front cover.

Lloyd Kahn, publisher, Shelter Publications and Jean Anderson, who granted permission for use of the stretching sketches on Hole #17.

John Turner, Mr. Nautilus, whose website (arthurjonesexercise.com) remains a fountain of information on high-intensity training and everything Arthur Jones. I value his friendship.

William E. Jones, son of Nautilus inventor Arthur Jones, who granted permission to quote from his father's work.

Arthur Jones, a master educator, forced people to think - often by a single question - and then lingered until they truly understood. A sincere display of interest in his subject frequently forced the Nautilus and MedX inventor to peel a thin layer from a tough façade. His ability to read people, communicate and motivate were by-products of his brilliance. Arthur backed strong opinions by fact and logic; but was first to admit that he sometimes did *not* know. A rare breed – sorely missed.

INTRODUCTION

The wood structure provided timely shelter from wind and rain. It featured three green walls laden with carvings from the past and an open side supported by a central beam - a *must-touch* to secure occupational status for the day. A stone's throw beyond was the golf shop framed by a stunning city skyline some eighty miles away, but rarely the focus. When the pro signaled, you had to be ready. One by one we were called to duty - a band of scruffy kids trying to make a buck.

Not an easy buck: The terrain was a succession of hills that posed as a ski resort during winter months. Two bags or a double loop would send you home weary - in our case, a mile or so.

But we were young ... and that view, magnificent.

The first tee of the Lookout Point Golf and Country Club in Fonthill, Ontario was perched on the highest point of the Niagara peninsula and featured a view of the spray from Niagara Falls to the east, and the Toronto skyline to the north. The course was commissioned for design in 1919 and completed in 1922 by Walter J. Travis who won the US Amateur in 1900, 1901 and 1903, and the British Amateur in 1904. Lookout Point hosted numerous provincial championships as well as the General Brock Open, a fixture on the PGA Tour in the 1930's. Steve Kozak, a former club-champion for whom I carried, caddied for Walter Hagan in the 1935 event. And Ben Hogan once won a long-drive contest from that same first tee. The club was most famous, however, for amateur sensation, Marlene Stewart Streit, Canada's single entry - to date - in the World Golf Hall of Fame.

At the time, we cared about one thing only: If we worked the weekend, we could play Monday morning. We never missed. One Monday, Rusty Kruty and I dodged the clubhouse to play sixty-three holes before *getting the boot* at sundown. My brother and I soon became junior members - and played and played. We were dumped at the doorstep in the morning and fetched in the evening, which did more than keep us off the streets. Al secured a golf scholarship at Austin Peay State University in Clarkesville, Tennessee - and I wasn't far behind. I captained the golf team at McMaster University in Hamilton, Ontario, where I earned Bachelor degrees in English and physical education.

Together we climbed the ranks at the club and earned a spot in the *Dirty Dozen* - an elite group of low-handicap golfers who played Saturday and Sunday mornings. The jump from caddy to elite was abrupt and, at times, awkward. I barely had a dime to throw in the pot and didn't drink. So, I sat at the 19th hole, sipping ginger ale and absorbing the play-by-play description and vivid language of the game, both good and bad. There was no shortage of entertainment on the hill.

The weekend master of ceremonies was a man who went out of his way to make Al and me welcome. Sam Balsom, the club jester, kept a cigar firmly in place during a swing that rotated a hairy, barrel-chest within a half-open shirt. His two-handicap dominated the course; his character governed beyond. Sam was louder than most - always had a story to top what was out there - and had the joint in stitches when he abandoned his chair to demonstrate the bizarre events of the day. It may have been my first exposure to golf performance, but it did little to endear him to the membership. The 19th hole was not hidden in the privacy of the men's locker room. Some were offended by the volume.

Sam hailed from nearby St. Catharines where he played a nine-hole course that was not on anyone's list. St David's, a 2,650-yard layout established on the outskirts of town near Queenston in 1910 by an architect who chose to remain anonymous, was nestled at the base of the Niagara escarpment – a long, cliff-like ridge of rock that ran westward from New York State through the Great Lakes to Illinois.

The escarpment made history; St. David's did not. In fact, every time Sam brought up the name, he took it on the chin. *"I took the big hitters - Mike 'the Krack,' 'Fiery,' Johnny Krow - out to St. David's,"* he declared one day to a less-than-sober audience, *"and they couldn't score."* The laughter triggered another round ... and aroused my curiosity.

Years after Sam's passing, I drove to St. David's to check it out. As warned - it was hard to find: Nine holes; two sets of tees; no clubhouse, practice facility or signage; and a shack of a pro shop. The course provided a pleasant walk but my one-under-par sixty-nine satisfied two curiosities: The anonymity of the architect, and the notion that Sam's long-hitting foursome must not have been *on* that day.

That would change.

I continued to *take on the big hitters* as I climbed golf's ladder – won a few club championships at Lookout, several collegiate events, a handful of invitational tournaments around the province and qualified for the Porter Cup at the Niagara Falls Country Club, Lewiston, New York, in 1973. There, I played with Bill Rogers (who won the British Open at Royal St. George's in 1981) and was followed by a threesome that included Craig Stadler and Gary Koch, and another that featured defending champion, Ben Crenshaw. My seventy-two did not stack up. Rogers shot sixty-six the first time he saw the course … and was disgusted with his play. I decided, then and there, that I would not eat peanut-butter sandwiches the rest of my life.

Plan B was prompted by another event that occurred around the time I first touched that green beam on the hill - a Christmas gift, a 110-pound set of barbells from Sears.*

At fourteen, I posted six Weider of Canada® charts on the wall in a corner of the basement - bodybuilding champions demonstrating exercises to convert skinny to athletic. I don't know how I survived. Some movements were exactly what you would expect from a Neanderthal - dangerous. But danger had purpose. As my play improved, I supplemented basic exercises from the charts with those of golf legend, Gary Player, for years swinging a heavy dumbbell with my left arm in an attempt to simulate the swing. Yet, I never became strong enough to swing the stripped-down barbell he demonstrated in his 1968 book, *Gary Player's Positive Golf.*

I moved south to pursue a Master's degree in physical education from the University of North Carolina at Greensboro, where weather provided year-round access to my passion. Upon graduation, I taught four years at Averett College (now, Averett University) in Danville, Virginia, where - among other duties - I established and coached the men's and women's varsity golf teams. That was followed by a four-year stint at high school in Caracas, Venezuela, where I formally entered the field of exercise by opening South

America's first Nautilus gym in 1980 – a venture that led to the preparation of that nation's male and female golf teams for the World Team Amateur Championship in 1986.

By then, my approach to training for sports had been shattered by an article written by Nautilus inventor, Arthur Jones. "Specificity in Strength Training ... The Facts and Fables," published in the *Athletic Journal* in May, 1977, clearly demonstrated that many of the exercises I had practiced for years would more likely hurt than help golf. The philosophical approach of my golf idol, Mr. Player, was also wrong for reasons related to a subject I had studied (but never learned) in 1968 - motor learning. Two glaring truths emerge from the study of how we learn movement skills:

1. *Specificity of skill exists.*
2. *Transfer of skill does not.*

Together they expose the nonsense that currently exists in the field of exercise as it relates to physical preparation for sports. *Performance Training*, as it is called, is not what it appears, and far from what experts would have you believe. Its commercial application is based upon false premises and grounded in the use of inferior equipment and training techniques, some outright dangerous. This time, danger to no purpose struck clear to the bone.

Physical preparation for golf has taken a sharp dogleg left and dragged a slew of enthusiasts in its wake. Traditional strength training and stretching have been replaced by "*the correction of faulty movement patterns*" through exercise – an approach designed to create a more *functional* outcome. It does not. The combination of strength training and skill training in an exercise setting compromises both. Arthur Jones said it best, "*BS is rather easy to establish, and once established, almost impossible to eradicate.*"

The philosophical approach and simple exercise guidelines of *Golf Performance Training ... What They Won't Tell You* will improve performance on the course in a way that movement-based training cannot. Of equal importance, it will identify what to avoid.

It's time to expose the truth ... to take on the big hitters *off* the course.

FRONT NINE

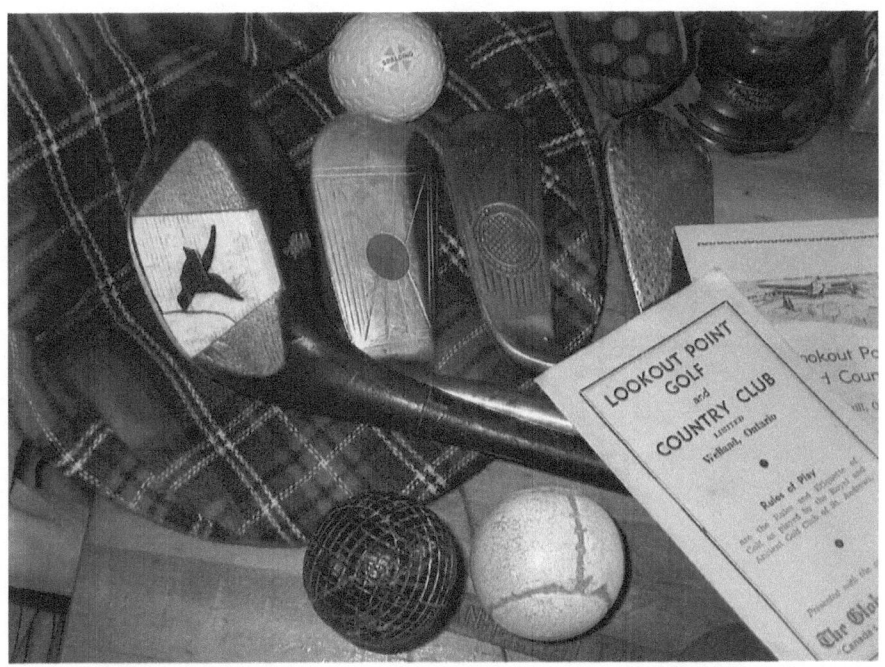

OUT

Hole #1: 423 Yards, Par 4

IMPROVING FUNCTIONAL ABILITY IN GOLF

In May of 1986, the Federacion Venezolana de Golf asked me to prepare a select group of male and female athletes for the World Team Amateur Championship to be held later that year at Lagunita Country Club on the outskirts of Caracas. At the time, I owned the largest Nautilus facility in town, had established a sound reputation, and was given ample time for a task I was honored to accept.

My first challenge was to sell the product – strength training - to a group of high-skilled non-believers, none of whom were actively involved in exercise. Fortunately, the Federation helped by twisting a few polo shirts and keeping strict attendance records throughout. In the end, only one team member - a 52-year-old male - quit after an early workout, deciding it was *not for him*. The younger players stayed the course and believed their efforts worthwhile. Workouts were based on Nautilus training principles - brief, hard, infrequent exercise – and performed on machines only, a far cry from today's approach.

By tournament's end, the host nation had performed admirably (Canada claimed the Eisenhower Trophy by a narrow margin over the United States). The Venezuelan Golf Federation acknowledged my efforts, and several athletes continued to exercise in my facility, the highest honor.

During the process, I was invited to contribute an article to the official publication of the championship, and submitted the following:

Improving Functional Ability in Golf

Functional ability in any sport is a product of five factors: bodily proportions, neurological efficiency, cardiovascular condition, skill and muscular strength. While all of these factors are important, the first two – bodily proportions, which provides muscles with an advantage in leverage, and neurological efficiency, which permits muscles to work at a higher level of efficiency - are genetic and not subject to change, good or bad. Attention should therefore focus on the final three improvable factors.

Cardiovascular ability is a requirement for life itself – and a lack of this ability may prevent a high level of performance. But no amount of cardiovascular ability can perform work. Movement is produced by the working muscles.

A high level of skill allows muscles to work more efficiently by channeling the force produced by them into a proper direction. But skill alone cannot produce movement.

Only the muscles produce movement, perform work, provide energy, and to a great extent, protect an athlete from injury. Muscle strength is the only productive factor; the others are supportive in nature.

Most golfers devote a large percentage of their training time to skill improvement, as they should, since skill may be the single most important factor in any sport. Some golfers additionally practice some form of cardiovascular exercise since at least a minimum is required in golf and because golf, under present-day conditions, may not provide that minimum. But few golfers ever do anything for their muscular strength. It is by far the most misunderstood factor, the most neglected factor, and yet is the only productive factor. And here we are in the final quarter of the twentieth century with thousands of athletes and coaches, golfers not excluded, who are literally afraid of their muscles, fearing that increased strength will somehow hurt their ability, slow them down, reduce their flexibility or otherwise limit their performance.

A champion in any sport is usually superior in all of the five factors, with perhaps one exception – his or her strength is seldom what it could be and almost never as high as it should be. And regardless of how large or small the role of strength plays in golf, performance will always be less than what it

4

could be if this factor is not addressed. And don't get me wrong. No amount of muscle will help an athlete if he lacks the skill to use it effectively – but no amount of muscle will hurt his skill either; instead, proper strength training will always improve his functional ability. It will make an athlete faster not slower, increase flexibility in any area of movement and increase cardiovascular conditioning, metabolic endurance and the athlete's ability to withstand injury.

The golf swing is a complex movement, making the brain's task of coordination difficult. But when the brain is given more efficient and powerful tools, that is, stronger muscles, it recruits a smaller number of muscle fibers to perform the task, making the coordination of all muscle groups used in that movement less complex.

How does one go about building strength for golf? Without becoming involved in a refutation of common misconceptions, the basic rules for proper exercise performed for the purpose of gaining strength can be stated very briefly: use full-range exercise to increase flexibility and develop strength over the entire length of the muscle; perform all movements in a slow fashion, avoiding sudden or jerky movements; continue all exercises to a point of momentary muscle failure, which point should be reached around 10-12 repetitions with as much resistance as possible; and perform all exercises in good form, never allowing form to deteriorate in an attempt to use more resistance or increase the number of repetitions.

If Nautilus machines are available, only one set of 10-12 repetitions is sufficient to provide very good results as long as each exercise is carried to the point of muscle failure in good form. With Nautilus equipment, a maximum of twelve exercises that involve the muscles used in golf should be performed. If free weights or Universal machines are available, two sets of exercise for each body part may be required for best results. In this case, sets for the same body part should not be done consecutively, and the total number of sets performed should not exceed twenty. Such a workout, properly performed with little or no rest between exercises, should last 20-25 minutes using Nautilus equipment or 30-35 minutes with free weights or Universal machines. Workouts should be performed three times per week on alternate days, preferably after one has played or practiced golf.

Do not make the common error of trying to repeat the movements of the golf swing or parts of it against resistance. Strength is general by nature and requires a maximum overload for proper development. Skill retention or development depends upon total specificity, that is, practice of the swing itself with the same tool in exactly the same manner, without an overload. The closer you come to specificity in exercise, the more you are likely to interrupt your skills. The two must remain separate. Therefore, build the muscles involved in golf in the most efficient and effective way you can without trying to be specific - without trying to duplicate the actions of the golf swing. Then learn to use that strength to your advantage in the only way possible, by practice of the golf swing itself. Anything else will hurt far more than it will help.

The missing link to improve functional ability in golf is proper strength training. Use it ... you have everything to gain and nothing to lose except problems. And while it certainly will not solve all of your problems, would it not be wise to settle for a solution to at least some of them?

That message was a far cry from what transpired in my basement throughout high-school and college, and a far cry from current efforts to train movement, rather than muscle.

Two facts are clear:

1. Only the strength of muscle contraction produces movement and performs work. The supporting cast - bodily proportions, neurological efficiency, cardiovascular ability and skill – assists the effort by providing leverage, range of motion, and a more efficient and effective outcome.
2. The trainable factors – muscle strength, cardiovascular ability and skill - can and should be improved in order to attain your athletic potential:
   - *Muscle strength* can be increased by progressive resistance exercise; in specific, proper strength training.
   - *Cardiovascular ability* can be improved by progressive aerobic exercise, or through proper strength training.
   - *Skill* can be improved by skill training alone.

Priorities

The establishment of training priorities is crucial to an efficient and effective result. In light of the discussion above, the acquisition of muscle strength - the *only* productive factor – appears to top the list, but does not. Golf is a high-skill sport, and skill deserves top billing:

Priority One: The skill component of golf is estimated to be as high as 90 percent, which doesn't leave room for much else - including exercise. Regardless of the actual percentage, the claim is strong: *The majority of a golfer's time and energy should be devoted to skill training - the development of a repetitive swing and a repertoire of effective short-game skills.*

I was introduced to the importance of skill the day I was paired with Toronto sensation, Ken Trowbridge in a junior tournament in the mid 1960's. Ken outdrove me by sixty yards on every hole – and flushed two years of strength training down the drain - with arms half my size. His club speed was generated by superior skill - leverage, timing and sequence. Years later, we were paired in an invitational tournament in Peterborough, Ontario with an identical outcome, notwithstanding that I had become stronger. As Arthur Jones stated, *"Some have it and some don't,"* and it was clear that I did not. Ken earned a golf scholarship at Indiana University and pursued a successful career as a professional, despite the loss of an eye in a bizarre golf-related accident.

A second exposure to the significance of skill occurred when I witnessed an exhibition by Moe Norman at the Canadian Junior Championship in 1965. The legend hit ball after ball - rapid-fire and dead straight - with no apparent effort. I witnessed the same on three subsequent occasions: At Lookout Point in a Pro-Pro Best-Ball tournament; at St. Georges (Toronto) in the 1968 Canadian Open; and at an exhibition in Orlando, Florida, a few years before he passed. *"Ladies and gentlemen,"* he began in Orlando, *"I'm the only man on the planet who can hit a golf ball straight every time I swing at it. That's not my opinion. It's the opinion of those who have seen me over the years. I'm going to hit five hundred balls this afternoon. If you see one crooked shot, stop and tell me ..."* He scanned a crowd of three hundred spectators surrounding the tee and added *"...because you won't."* Midway through, Moe was asked how he got so good. *"I hit five hundred balls a day for forty years,"* he replied. Rumor had the number at more, but the point remains: It took a lot of skill training to achieve a level of proficiency that many called *the best ball-striker ever.* Golf Digest® magazine analyzed his swing (December, 1995) and described it *as close to the machine as we have ever seen.* Moe's contemporaries believed he could *not* hit a golf ball off-line (because he never did); and Tiger Woods once commented, *"There are only two players who truly 'owned their swings', Ben Hogan and Moe Norman."* I never saw Hogan, but I saw Moe Norman – *Golf's Greatest Show on Earth.*

Skill proficiency is not a matter of hitting more balls than the next guy: It involves perfecting a motion that produces optimum results. Ironically, neither Ben Hogan nor Moe Norman took a formal lesson. Both dug their talent *out of the dirt* without much in the way of external assistance. In contrast, today's top professionals tow an entourage – a swing coach, short game guru, physical trainer and psychologist – in an effort to reach the same end, and no one's got there yet.

While perfection may never be attained in the game, skill is trainable - and time spent in that direction is crucial to success.

Priority Two: Strength, the only productive and trainable factor that contributes to functional ability, should be your second priority. Increasing the strength of the muscles used in the various skills of golf goes a long way to enhance proficiency and protect you from injury.

Priority Three: Superior cardiovascular ability may assist those who walk a hilly course, or frequently stray from the beaten path. It can also make you feel ready to play and boost confidence. But in the end, its contribution is minimized by the fact that a leisurely stroll on a flat course, or riding around in a golf cart, can hardly be defined as *aerobic.*

Trial and Error

My start in golf came from a man who stepped from the pro-shop door – the door that faced the caddy shack on top of the hill - into the Ontario Golf Hall of Fame as a teaching professional. As he had with Marlene Stewart Streit and others, Gordon McInnis Sr. taught me how to grip the club, position the ball in relation to my feet, assume proper posture, take proper aim, and more importantly, to *swing* the club. What more could I ask? It was up to me to piece the puzzle together.

A swing that repeats requires specificity, replication and constant correction to etch an effective pattern in the neuromuscular system. Everything has to be *exactly* the same – the input, the timing and the sequence. The flight of the ball and accompanying physical sensations led me to detect and correct swing flaws for the next effort as my body became proficient at sensing what was *different*.

The sensory input involved in any physical movement is specific. *Any change of any element* that has been established through repetition is deemed an intrusion, subject to its own interpretation. The interpretation of dissimilar information results in a dissimilar output - in effect, a different skill. How long does it take to adjust to the feel of a new set of clubs, or effect a swing change suggested by a professional? Practicing golf with a modification detectable by the sensory system is akin to practicing a new and different skill, and *different* means non-specific to the task.

To clarify, would you practice tennis to improve skill at golf? Not likely. Yet, this is exactly what happens when the focus of golf training shifts to movement, rather than to the muscles that produce movement.

Let's examine, in greater detail, the process of trial and error.

Hole #2: 135 Yards, Par 3

SKILL ACQUISITION

I n the 1960's, I studied a subject that has long been ignored in the field of exercise - motor learning. A basic understanding of *how we learn movement skills* first requires the definition of confusing terms: *skill* and *ability*.

A *skill* is a specific movement you learn - climbing stairs, throwing a baseball, combing your hair, roller skating or chipping a ball in golf. Some skills (like walking) are part of a general motor program and require no conscious thought; others require frequent, specific practice and plenty of thought. The ideal in any performance is to execute with little or no conscious effort, which is why - through practice - some can make the performance of a golf skill look easy.

Abilities are underlying traits that support skill performance. In broad physical terms, abilities include: Strength, power, speed, cardiovascular endurance, flexibility, agility, coordination and balance. Their activation results in fundamental actions that take place without direct or conscious control. Properly linked, they determine how well motor skills are performed from a general perspective.

Some abilities are trainable, while others are not:

> *Strength, power and speed* are limited by genetic potential, but can be enhanced by greater muscle-mass and skill proficiency.

> *Cardiovascular endurance and flexibility* are limited by genetic potential, but can be increased through training specifics.

> *Agility, coordination and balance* are determined by genetics, and *not* subject to change.[1]

To be clear:

- *Skill* is the movement itself, the motor task, the output.
- A*bility* is a background trait that supports skill, but does not provide specific movement patterns.

The contribution of a general ability to a skill varies from task to task. Skill A, for example, may feature the ability to balance with less emphasis on speed or endurance, while Skill B may require the opposite. The unique requirements of the abilities involved from one skill to another support the following:

- That each skill is unique.
- That proficiency in one skill does not ensure proficiency in another.
- That practice of one skill has no influence on the proficiency of another skill. For example, an individual may possess the ideal combination of abilities to be proficient in Skill A, but lack the perfect mix for Skill B.

Confusion occurs when similar abilities, such as balance or agility, underlie the performance of two *different* skills, which leads to belief in a crossover of skills. Not so. Abilities may flow freely from one skill to another, but the skill of one task *does not* crossover or transfer to the skill of another.

How We Learn

There are four stages of information processing that define motor learning and skill refinement: Identification of the stimulus via sensory perception – the input; selection of an appropriate response; programming of the motor system to produce the desired movement and complete the task; and the output, which may or may not achieve the intended goal.

Let's examine each stage to see what golfers face.

Input

Input during the learning process and memory retrieval is based on sensory perception – what can be seen, heard, tasted, smelled, and touched. The feedback from these sensors delivers a unique set of instructions to the brain to control movement according to the specific goals of the task. In golf, the major sensory information is transmitted via the following:

- Muscle spindles, located between muscle fibers, sense muscle length and help determine the position and velocity of body parts.
- Golgi tendon organs, located at muscle-tendon junctions, provide information about muscle tension - reducing it, when necessary, to prevent injury.
- Joint receptors, located within the joint capsules, indicate the position of the joint. Their role in movement has yet to be determined.
- Cutaneous receptors, located in the skin, process information about touch and pressure.

All sensors work together to indicate body position, maintain equilibrium and establish movement patterns. The system compares the information it receives during movement to feedback it expects to receive, and makes adjustments based on what it perceives as the most efficient path to complete the task. When movement is slow, refinement takes place *on the go*. When movement is fast, as during a golf swing, proper form must be established *before* - and mistakes corrected *after* - the event.

Response

The body sorts through the incoming information to determine an appropriate response and produce a desired action – a process that improves with practice. Initially, the learning process is rife with physical and mental problem-solving, inconsistent input and outcome, inefficient movement patterns, errors, indecision, muscle tension and poor timing or execution. As skills improve, the individual becomes more relaxed, certain and decisive - and movement more efficient, fluid, accurate and automatic. The final output depends on prior experiences, motivation and individual ability.

Programming

During the learning process, the mind integrates the sensory information with the motor components it intends to use, creating a *blueprint* that makes each activity unique. The blueprint is used only if execution of the intended action is *exactly the same* as that of the blueprint. If the action varies or the blueprint is altered, the new information must be processed, compared to what is known and undergo its own learning process – essentially, establish a new blueprint. Therefore, regardless of how skills appear to be similar, one skill can have *no* direct or positive effect on another.

Output

The result of a specific input, response and program blueprint is a specific output - each task or skill is as unique as its feedback and programming. Consequently, the nature of one task is *non-specific* to another - and any attempt to enhance a skill by the performance of a seemingly similar but different skill is, as Arthur Jones often said, *"Useless for its intended purpose."*

As true as it is, the message has been ignored by those who promote *functional* and *sport-specific* training in the field of exercise, both of which are movement-oriented and violate the two bedrock principles of motor learning: Specificity and transfer.

Specificity

The article that first caught my attention (mentioned in the Introduction) was published in the *Athletic Journal*, (May, 1977): "Specificity in Strength Training ... The Facts and Fables." Nautilus inventor, Arthur Jones hit hard and fast.

> *Don't be misled ... and you might be on the subject of specificity.*
>
> *There are no degrees to specificity ... either you have it or you don't. A movement is utterly specific, or it isn't specific at all.*
>
> *This being true, as it is, it obviously follows that the only possible way to produce specificity in anything is by performing the act itself. In effect, the only possible specific training for basketball is the act of playing basketball ... the only possible specific training for swimming is swimming itself, and so on.*

Strength is general, and contributes to any activity ... but the applied demonstration of strength is specific; and learning to apply your strength properly in any activity requires skill training. Which skill training can come from only one possible source, the practice of the sport itself.[2]

Yet, this is what I hear in gyms on a daily basis ...

- *"Get into a golf stance during every exercise."*
- *"That's exactly how your backswing should feel."*
- *"This will increase your power at impact."*

... and what I've seen for decades:

- Drills and exercises that replicate some facet of the golf swing in an attempt to reinforce or strengthen the movement pattern itself.
- Attempts to rationalize lousy exercise behavior under the guise of *golf.*

Modern trainers believe that the traditional process of strengthening muscles is not sufficient. Muscles must be strengthened, they claim, *as they move in a manner and direction that best replicates how they are to be used*, which makes an interesting assumption: Muscles strengthened by traditional means may find themselves *unprepared* when called upon. Strength and its proper application, they say, must be acquired *at the same time* – a concept Jones called "*hogwash:*"

> *An exercise that is NEARLY specific will simply mess up your skills ... an exercise that is ALMOST specific will have the same bad result. So don't try to be specific in your exercises ... doing so is impossible in any case, and the closer you come the greater the danger of hurting your skill.*

> *Build strength in the best way possible ... with little or absolutely no regard to how that strength is to be used; then learn to use that strength to your greatest advantage in the only way possible, by practice of the sport itself.*[3]

Skill acquisition demands *specific* practice. The alteration of any element of a movement establishes a new and different motor program - the selection of new and different pathways, a *non-specific* skill. This is why a golf lesson may temporarily disrupt proficiency. And why golfers often comment on what they felt *after* the fact – "I lifted my head," "I kept weight on my back foot." When something feels *different*, body sensors inform - and the nervous system must process the *new* information.

Without question, the body senses a *difference* when resistance is applied to a skill movement. The change of speed or force imposed upon the working muscles creates confusion in the nervous system that may lead to an adverse outcome - precisely what occurs in today's approach to golf performance training.

Transfer

Transfer of skill refers to the attainment or loss of proficiency in a skill as a result of practicing a different skill. According to founder and former president of the International Association of Resistance Trainers (IART), Brian Johnston, "*It has been demonstrated time and again that positive transfer* (a positive outcome in reference to neuromuscular patterning, or skill) *is either non-existent or quite negligible (negligible among tasks that are almost exactly the same, but slightly different in some regard).*"[4]

The result of a specific stimulus is a specific response. Implementation of a motor pattern that is *nearly* similar or *completely dissimilar* does not have a positive influence on the performance of the target skill. The same applies to most underlying abilities. There is *no* correlation, for example, among activities that require balance. If a person cannot swing a golf club due to a balance issue, the problem *cannot* be improved by use of a balance board or Swiss ball. Any improvement in balance as a result of such action is confined to the skill of using that tool. *Balance is specific to the task and improves as skill improves.*[5] Attempts to improve balance during the golf swing should be addressed *during* the golf swing. A general application of *balance* training will *not* improve the balance component of a specific skill.

Can you improve your skill at golf by taking a racquetball lesson, or something *like* a golf lesson? No. You take a golf lesson. Yet, movement-based trainers continue to introduce clients to *new and different* movement skills, claiming that they will improve the performance of the *old*. Good luck.

False positive transfer

Despite the fact that positive transfer does *not* exist in skill training as illustrated above, many athletes report improved performance when they modify their workout routines from a traditional to a movement-based or skill-based structure (such as *functional* or *golf-specific* training). This may be due to one or more of the following:

- Increased motivation on the new system, for whatever reason(s), including the quality of coaching and the perception of a more-targeted approach.
- Better recovery from prior, lengthy periods of intense strength training, since skill-based exercises are less intense by design.
- Different styles of training.
- Nutritional modifications.
- Improved practice of the skills themselves.
- Individual maturation (the athlete becomes more capable within his or her means).

Other factors merit consideration:

- The reported improvement may have been achieved by other means in less time.
- Many athletes combine training modalities making it difficult to determine cause and effect.
- There are as many successful athletes who do *not* perform skill-based exercise as those who do.

Negative Transfer

Negative transfer occurs when learning one skill negatively affects the quality of another - when practice of a similar skill alters an existing motor pattern. According to Arthur Jones, the closer the new skill is to the old, the more likely the interference. For the most part, negative transfer is minimal (particularly if the old skills have been well ingrained), and more likely to surface during early developmental stages.

Facts related to the transfer of skill are clear …

- With *unlike* activities, there is no positive transfer, and probably no negative transfer.
- With *like* activities, there is no positive transfer, but a greater probability of negative transfer.

Skill-based advocates believe otherwise - that positive transfer exists with *like* and *unlike* activities - and they rarely acknowledge the existence of negative transfer.

Literature and Research

What does motor-learning literature and research reveal about specificity and transfer?

(1) From Richard A. Schmidt, PhD. *A common misconception is that fundamental abilities (reaction time, movement speed, flexibility, explosive strength and gross-body coordination) can be trained through various drills or other activities. The thinking is that, with some stronger ability, the athlete will see gains in performance for tasks with this underlying ability. For example, athletes are often given quickening exercises, with the hope that these exercises would train some fundamental ability to be quick, allowing quicker responses in their particular sport. Coaches often use various balancing drills to increase general balancing ability, eye movement exercises to improve vision, and many others. Such attempts to train fundamental abilities may sound fine, but usually they simply do not work. Time, and often money, would be better spent practicing the eventual goal skills.*

There are two correct ways to think of these principles. First, there is no general ability to be quick, to balance, or to use vision. Rather, quickness, balance, and vision are each based on many diverse abilities, so there is no single quickness ability, for example, that can be trained. Second, even if there were such general abilities, these are, by definition, genetic and not subject to modification through practice. Therefore, attempts to modify abilities with nonspecific drills are ineffective. A learner may acquire additional skill at the drill (which is a skill itself), but this learning does not transfer to the main skill of interest.[6]

(2) *Practice of non-specific coordination or quickening tasks will not produce transfer to specific sport skills. In regards to quickening exercises that involve many rapid skillful movements, transfer of learning is highly specific and occurs only when the practiced movements are identical.[7]*

(3) *Minor alterations from an exact action change the characteristics of the systems that produce the altered action. Such changes are potentially harmful to a well-trained athlete.[8]*

(4) *When training has occurred through participation in large-muscle total-body activities, such as running, rowing or Olympic lifting, there can be partial but minor transfer of training effects to simpler activities. For example, aerobic improvements derived from running (a complex activity) have been shown to produce improvements in the aerobic work of cycling (a simpler activity where the work occurs in fewer large muscle groups). The amount of transfer is marginal at best. The aerobic benefits that could be derived from one hundred hours of endurance running might translate into the equivalent effect of ten hours of endurance training for cycling. It would seem to be more expedient and economical to just train for ten hours on a bicycle rather than perform ten times as much running-training to get an improvement in cycling. As well, cycling produces specific endurance effects plus other associated benefits (which would not result from relying on the transfer of the running-training phenomenon).[9]*

(5) *Activities which look similar, but are performed at slightly different speeds, are most likely to be completely dissimilar in their training effects. Every alteration of path of movement or apparatus used is a different neuromuscular pattern of movement development.[10]*

When you alter the components of a skill, you create a unique and separate entity: Specificity of skill exists; transfer of skill does not ... as illustrated by the following:

Observations

When I was eight years old, Dad took me to Fort Erie, Ontario, to see a man who became my first sports hero. Eddie Feigner, the pitching sensation of a four-man softball team that barnstormed the country as *The King and his Court*, could make the ball curve left and right, dive *about two feet* and rise - at a time *the riser* was considered impossible. He pitched between his legs, from his knees, behind his back, from center field, from second base, blindfolded – all with the same result: Few saw it, and fewer hit it.

In a televised exhibition at Dodger Stadium in 1964, Feigner faced six of the best hitters in baseball: Willy Mays, Willy McCovey, Maury Wills, Harmon Killebrew, Roberto Clemente and Frank Robinson. Pitching from a softball distance of forty-six feet, he struck all of them out in a row – a classic example of the principles of motor learning at work. The hitters, without doubt, were highly skilled and possessed exceptional underlying abilities (hand-eye coordination, balance, timing, etc.) They were accustomed to pitches of all shapes and sizes but not to the shorter delivery distance, larger ball and faster pitching speed (Feigner was clocked at 104 miles per hour). The differences combined to create a non-specific skill. As similar as the tasks seemed, it was like asking a soccer goalkeeper to shoot skeet. The big hitters couldn't hit Feigner - the skill and ability requirements were different. There was *no* transfer of batting skill from baseball to softball.

My track and field instructor at McMaster University, Peter Radford from Great Britain, set a world record in 1960 for the 220-yard dash at 20.5 seconds. Since then, I have watched many 100-meter finals – from the great Russian sprinters; through Canada's single embarrassment, Ben Johnson; to the exploits of Jamaica's, Usain Bolt. The greats fall into one of two categories: those quick off the blocks, and those who are great closers. Quick off the blocks indicates *reaction* time (how quickly one reacts to the sound of the starting gun). Closing refers to *movement time* (how quickly one completes the task). Research on reaction and movement time shows no direct correlation between the two. Some athletes explode off the blocks in a sprint, only to lose to someone with greater movement-time ability. Research also shows no direct correlation between reaction time and movement time *within* the same individual. That is, increasing reaction-time ability does not enhance movement-time ability in any proportionate way - evidence that practicing a specific skill or ability is *not* likely to enhance another.

For two seasons, I assisted the Douglas High-School varsity baseball team in Parkland, Florida with their strength training. One day, by error, I walked into the office of the football coach who was immersed in a video that demonstrated the proper form of a competitive weight-lifting technique and football staple – the power clean. Most coaches (and strength coaches) believe that the power clean is one of the most *functional* exercises for football, contributing to a lineman's explosive ability on the field – an obvious belief in transfer. From a strength perspective, the power clean may contribute to success in football; but from a skill perspective it does not. If the power clean affects explosive movement off the line as much as they believe, then explosive movement off the line must affect the power clean to the same degree. Which means, players could stop performing the skill of exploding off the line and not lose efficiency because they have been performing power cleans in the gym. Good luck with that.

Last winter, I pulled into the parking lot of a public driving-range in North Palm Beach, Florida, in time to witness what was once considered a factor in the decline of the Roman Empire, but now enjoys universal acceptance. I parked in an advantageous spot and watched it unfold. *Act One* featured a fifteen year-old female destined for the tour – big bag, bright clothing and nice swing - accompanied by a man I called *The Juggler*. They stood eight feet apart, face-to-face and tossed tennis balls to each other in an obvious exhibition of hand-eye coordination. *Act Two* featured the young lady slowly swinging a golf club while standing on a pair of independent air-filled balance pads. Both acts were plucked from the archives of *functional* or movement-based training and represented obvious attempts to increase hand-eye coordination and balance, but the facts claim otherwise. Hand-eye coordination and balance are underlying *abilities* that are fully developed at an early age, and *not* subject to change or transfer. In plain

English, unless the teen plans to enter juggling competitions or lug a pair of balance pads to the first tee, the activities are useless. Furthermore, success at either remains specific to the task. That is, training a general concept of balance or hand-eye coordination does *not* ensure that either will improve when applied to *another* task that involves these abilities, in this case, golf. Perceived improvement remains with the practiced skill and represents another example of telling the world what they want to hear, rather than what occurs.

Conclusion

The study of motor learning reveals two glaring truths related to the acquisition of skill:

1. *Specificity of skill exists.*
2. *Transfer of skill does not.*

With that, the basic elements of proper skill training have been exposed. The holes that follow focus on the role of exercise in performance, and ultimately reveal the difference(s) between proper skill training and proper strength training.

References

1. Brian Johnston, *System Analysis* (Sudbury, ON: Bodyworx Publishing, 2001), 142.
2. Arthur Jones, "Specificity in Strength Training ... The Facts and Fables," *Athletic Journal*, May (1977).
3. Arthur Jones, "Specificity in Strength Training ... The Facts and Fables," *Athletic Journal*, May (1977).
4. Brian Johnston, *System Analysis* (Sudbury, ON: Bodyworx Publishing, 2001), 129.
5. Richard A. Schmidt, *Motor Learning and Performance: From Principles to Practice* (Champagne, IL: Human Kinetics Books, 1991).

6. Richard A. Schmidt, *Motor Learning and Performance: From Principles to Practice* (Champagne, IL: Human Kinetics Books, 1991), 222.

7. G.W. Sage, *An Introduction to Motor-Behavior: A Neuropsychological Approach* (Philippines: Addison-Wesley, 1971), 357.

8. B.S. Rushall and F.S. Pyke, *Training for Sports and Fitness* (Melbourne, Australia: Macmillan of Australia, 1991).

9. B.S. Rushall, "A Summary of Specificity," *Coaching Science Abstracts* 1, no. 2 (1992).

10. B.S. Rushall and F.S. Pyke, *Training for Sports and Fitness* (Melbourne, Australia: Macmillan of Australia, 1991), 77.

Hole #3: 483 Yards, Par 5

THE POTENTIAL BENEFITS OF EXERCISE

Osmael Sosa, the *King* of beauty pageants in Venezuela, entered my exercise facility in 1986 soliciting aid in the preparation of Miss Venezuela, Barbara Palacios, for the upcoming Miss Universe contest. He was quick to unveil a series of photos that, in his opinion, limited her chance of success. *"As is,"* he proclaimed, pointing to her defects, *"she will not win Miss Universe."* Most would have taken her *"As is,"* but I had a few questions:

"How long do we have to achieve the goal?"

"One month and five days," he replied.

The conversation came to a halt. I was not a surgeon.

Mr. Sosa did not bring her in next day, as promised; but Miss Palacios won the pageant a month later, *without* exercise. ... So much for experts.

Fortunately, that was not the case with the Venezuelan Golf Federation.

The process of preparing the national teams for international competition that same year involved marketing the potential benefits of exercise to assure participants that strength training would not *screw up* their skill. Fortunately, the six-month window proposed by the Federation allowed time to overcome the initial shock of training - vital in a sport where a single swing can derail a program. The sell wasn't easy, but did not change the facts.

Proper exercise can provide the following benefits:

1. An increase in muscle strength.
2. An increase in flexibility.
3. An increase in cardiovascular condition.
4. An improvement in body composition (more muscle, less fat).
5. A decrease in the possibility of injury.

Let's examine the contribution of each to the Royal and Ancient game.

Strength

Muscle strength is more important to golf than most imagine. First and foremost, the strength of muscle contraction is the only thing (from the list above) that produces movement. Without it, there is no swing, no walk, no chip, no putt - no golf.

How can strength contribute to a high-skill sport such as golf? Arthur Jones provided a launching pad. *"Short of checkers and chess,"* he claimed, *"a stronger athlete is a better athlete."*

1. Strength is a major component in golf's power equation: It increases the potential to generate club-head speed, which results in more distance.
2. The force requirement of golf-related efforts is determined by the nervous system. An increase in muscle strength facilitates the execution of a skill – by less effort and physiological cost - which increases the muscle's reserve for future efforts. Greater muscle strength opens the door to greater muscle endurance.
3. Strength acquired through proper training is the gateway to all of the other potential benefits:
   - It can vastly increase flexibility,
   - Is the limiting factor in cardiovascular efficiency,
   - Is the key to increasing and sustaining a high metabolic rate and low body-fat,
   - And is crucial to the prevention of injury.
4. Golf is neither checkers nor chess.

Despite evidence to support the relationship of strength to performance, many of the finest golfers on the planet refuse to do anything about their strength – the risk is too great. *"If golf is 90 percent skill and 10 percent strength,"* they rationalize, *"why bother?"* The answer is simple: If you fail to reach your strength potential – fill in the 10 percent - you fail to reach your performance potential.

If a muscle is called upon to contract with 10 percent of its maximum force at a specific moment during the golf swing, a stronger muscle contributes a greater force input than a weaker muscle:

- 10 percent of one hundred units of force = ten units of force
- 10 percent of two hundred units of force = twenty units of force

And if the task of filling that request is diminished by increased strength, the working muscles possess a greater reserve for future efforts, which favorably affects practice frequency and duration, as well as fatigue during the final holes of play. Once again:

- 10 percent of one hundred units of force = ten units of force + ninety units of reserve
- 10 percent of two hundred units of force = twenty units of force + one hundred and eighty units of reserve

Another point deserves mention: Regardless of strength level, your body does *not* allow itself to use *all* of its strength. Most muscles, during non-emergency conditions, recruit approximately 30 percent of their available fibers during a maximum effort. Seventy percent will *not* participate due to safety concerns: If a muscle is allowed to recruit *all* of its fibers (as during an emergency or electrocution), bones break. Some individuals can recruit 50 percent of their fibers during an all-out effort; others, only 10 percent. Regardless, the body's ability to recruit muscle fibers is genetic and *not* subject to change.

From a skill perspective, golfers rarely employ a maximum effort, unless to get out of heavy rough. But it's nice to know that strength is there, when needed. From a strength perspective, if the body perceived the swing as an emergency - or a three-foot putt as an electrocution (as it sometimes feels) – you'd surely break more than the course record.

...Too Strong?

Can you be too strong for golf? No one can answer with certainty, but observations can be made. Television interviews and articles generally reflect a conservative approach to strength training among the game's elite: A fear of lifting weights still exists. The majority who commit to exercise perform cardiovascular activity and stretching to keep pace with peers, but most are reluctant to perform large-muscle, progressive resistance training with any fervor. *"I do a little bit of strength training,"* said PGA Tour player Justin Leonard in a Golf Digest® interview. *"I don't want to look like a linebacker."* Don't worry. Most men can't build muscles to a size that would impede a golf swing, with few exceptions...

A Venezuelan orthopedic surgeon with whom I played in the 1980's performed twenty years of bodybuilding *before* he took up the game. His massive chest allowed bent-arm-only access to the club from the sides, limiting his ability to generate speed - something we never discussed.

I was once paired with a man who was a cross between Ben Hogan and Hulk Hogan, but not a golfer. Formally introduced as *"Canada's Bench Press Champion,"* he was all over the lot. When he finally hit a fairway, I had to wave him aside for safety. We spent most of the day looking for balls, which left a single impression – was all that muscle harmful to his game?

I think not. Neither man (above) possessed the skill necessary to excel at golf. One lacked the time; the other, the interest. Yet, they were both better off strong and healthy than not.

If an athlete with superior golf skills possessed an advanced level of strength, you would literally have superman on the links. Tiger Woods comes to mind – an elite athlete with the drive and work ethic to achieve his skill and strength potentials. In his heyday, competitors stood still as he flew by, which turned heads in the right direction, including that of Rory McIlroy.

Flexibility

I currently work with a population of aging golfers who toot the same horn: *"I need more distance,"* *"I can't make a full turn."* Solutions are numerous:

lighter equipment, increased muscle strength and/or flexibility, and decreased body fat. Like their professional superiors, most balk at the idea of initiating a full-blown strength program. They prefer an equipment upgrade or any activity related to flexibility - stretching, yoga, Pilates or gyrotonics. Can you blame them?

The acquisition of flexibility, the ability to move through a greater range of motion, represents an easy solution – but not the most effective for golf. Increasing a backswing turn through enhanced flexibility creates its own problems. In theory, a greater coil results in greater torque and club-head speed at impact. But, increasing the length of a backswing by superior coil means that the club travels a greater distance, both up and down. And while the added length may translate into greater speed at impact, it means that timing the hit must change – a process that could take months to refine. A longer swing also creates more time and distance for error to rear its ugly head. How many golfers, including the elite, control the direction of their ball more effectively with shorter (*versus* longer) clubs and swings? The longer the distance a club travels, the greater the potential for control problems.

A friend from Jupiter Hills, Florida, once shared two sayings from an old Scottish pro at Royal Dornoch:

- *"Don't be concerned about the backswing. You're not hitting in that direction anyway."*
- *"I've shortened many a swing, laddie, but can't recall ever lengthening one."*

Think twice about adding length to your backswing by means of flexibility exercises.

The majority of golf performance programs target inflexibility as a major limiting factor in the execution of a proper swing. I disagree. While it might be so in some instances, only an extreme case would cripple success. To illustrate: Trainers commonly target tight hamstrings (which most golfers have) and point to the role they play in interfering with proper posture at address. True. But the tightness would have to be extreme to negatively affect your ability to assume a proper stance. Another example: A tight soleus muscle, located below the calf in the lower leg, limits your ability to bend at the knee and assume a proper golf posture. Once again, the tightness would have to be extreme to produce a negative outcome.

On the other side of the coin, increased flexibility has benefits that rarely enter the conversation. *One*: It makes you feel loose, which leads to a relaxed sensation as you play – a good thing. *Two*: It may protect you from injury by reducing stress on muscles when they approach their range-of-motion limits. In this regard, stretching must be accompanied by strengthening. Injury is ultimately determined by the strength - not the flexibility - of a muscle/joint system *versus* the amount of force applied to it. You can control the former, but not the latter.

Joint flexibility must be accompanied by adequate muscle strength to control movement and prevent injury.

...Too Flexible?

Twenty years ago, I helped design and implement a golf training program in Jupiter, Florida. To everyone's delight, the program shot out of the blocks, attracting PGA, LPGA and Champions Tour professionals, as well as local amateurs. One young man who played on the Golden Bear Tour, Jeff Street, displayed an extreme range of motion during stretching exercises that served him well. Jeff won three consecutive events that year, plus the end-of-season money-title. His success - with due respect - was more related to his skill than flexibility. Jeff would never use the full potential of his range of motion during any part of a golf swing.

Two-time LPGA winner, Jackie Gallagher Smith, demonstrated a similar capacity for flexibility. Like Jeff, however, she would never use that degree of motion during play.

Both Jeff and Jackie had the skill and strength to control the range of motion necessary for the task at hand - rarely the case with the average player. Many female golfers, for example, possess the flexibility to create a full swing, but lack the strength to control it. The momentum of the backswing, in many cases, takes them to positions beyond *ideal*, which may lead to weight-distribution and balance issues.

Flexibility can be increased by performing a brief series of simple stretching exercises as outlined on Hole #17. It can also be attained through proper strength training.

Most golfers do not associate flexibility with strength gain. In fact, the two are viewed as opposites: Strength-building exercise contracts or shortens muscles, while flexibility movements lengthen them. Assuming proper form and execution, the process of strengthening requires a muscle to return to its starting position to perform another repetition. It is *during* the return – the lowering of the resistance and lengthening of the muscle - that flexibility can be increased.

Three factors affect the outcome: The quality of resistance, the quantity of resistance and the speed at which the resistance approaches the muscle's extension limit.

The Quality of Resistance

The stimulus for flexibility increase during strength training occurs when sensors within muscle tendons feel *tension* (a force or resistance) near their limit of extension. But force or resistance alone is not enough to trigger the appropriate response. It must be *the correct dosage* of resistance applied *at the correct angle* – both of which depend on the choice of exercise tools.

Free-weight exercises, with few exceptions, provide little or no resistance when a muscle reaches an extended position. The start position of a standing biceps curl, for example, provides no resistance or force to extended biceps tendons because gravity is parallel to the direction of the tendons, instead of at 180° to the tendon's direction of pull. Pulley stations suffer the same dilemma – the applied force often pulls in a direction that does not directly oppose that of the working muscle. If there is no force or tension properly applied to a muscle in extension, there is no stretch. The only tool that satisfies the requirement for flexibility increase during progressive resistance exercise is a single-joint machine with a proper cam. It applies a correct amount of resistance - at 180° to the pull of the muscle - throughout a full range-of-motion.

Unfortunately, quality machines are scarce. Today's manufacturers make few single-axis exercise stations due to decreased demand, and some produce lousy equipment. To add, trainees often make poor equipment choices during exercise or fail to perform movements through a full range-of-motion – both of which influence the potential for flexibility gains.

The Quantity of Resistance

Stretching is generally performed without external assistance. That is, the weight of the body part or limb that the target muscle moves becomes the resistance. External assistance (provided by a stretching rope, towel or training partner) can make the applied resistance more effective. So, too can the added resistance of progressive strength training, as follows:

> *Place your upper arm, palm up, on a table so that your elbow is on the top edge of the table and your forearm is fully extended beyond. Maintain that position a few minutes and allow gravity to stretch the biceps tendons. The weight of your forearm provides the resistance to create the desired result.*

> *Repeat the process with a small weight in your hand. Now your biceps tendons will stretch to their limit (within the confines of the joint system) in less time. Gravity has a greater effect working against a greater resistance. The same occurs during exercise, where - given a proper tool and a full range-of-motion – a progressive resistance can expedite the stretching process.*

Speed of Movement

Proper form is crucial to flexibility gains *during* exercise. Working muscles *must move slowly* as they approach a position of full extension to allow them to relax and elongate. A rapid or jerky lowering of resistance as a muscle approaches its movement limits activates a physiological response called a *stretch reflex*, a contraction to counter what the body perceives as impending danger. When that occurs, flexibility gains are nullified.

Efficient and effective flexibility increases can occur *during* strength training by using proper form and quality equipment. The flexibility gains produced during *Project Total Conditioning*, an exercise experiment outlined on Hole #13, provide statistical proof.

Cardiovascular Condition

In general terms, cardiovascular or aerobic ability is defined as the delivery of oxygen from the heart and lung systems to the working muscles, and its role in sports is well documented. Cardiovascular capacity is commonly defined by heart rate and developed by sustaining or surpassing a minimum rate (*defined by age*) for a period of time (*a minimum of approximately fifteen minutes*) at regular intervals (*two or three times a week*).

Under those guidelines, golf can barely be called aerobic. The mandatory use of golf carts around the country has all but destroyed the cardiovascular value of a brisk walk with a set of clubs over your shoulder, not to mention the caddy industry.

Nonetheless, a sound cardiovascular capacity has benefits that apply to golf. At fourteen, I started training for golf by running and lifting weights, and soon developed a high level of aerobic condition that proved useful. Young and strong, I boldly stood on the putting green - between the caddy shack and pro shop - convinced that my out-of-shape competitors could *not* beat me under any circumstances. At a more mellow age, I walked mountain courses where sustained climbs left me out of breath on the next tee. A superior cardiovascular capacity improved my ability to recover between efforts, retarded fatigue during the final holes, allowed play at my pace, and elevated my confidence. It left no regrets.

In 1975, I won the 12th Annual Glen Eagle Classic in Bolton, Ontario after sleeping in my car the night before in the back of a church parking lot (to my Mother's delight) and after running seven miles two hours before tee time. My seventy-three edged out the recently-crowned Ontario Amateur champion by a shot - which should have motivated him to join me on my next outing. Unfortunately, the event was not awarded major status.

Despite my steadfast pursuit of fitness, the man who taught me the game did not believe in the value of aerobic training. *"Every time you get over the ball to putt,"* he insisted, *"you're still huffing and puffing from all the running you do."* And that included a few runs to the course. It was the *only* thing he said that I ignored.

A superior cardiovascular capacity contributes to any athletic endeavor and can be acquired through traditional means (swim, run, bike; a brisk treadmill walk, a stepper) or through sustained large-muscle activity, including proper strength training.

Body Composition

...Like a Dream

In 1972, I stood on the clubhouse porch of the Sedgefield Country Club in Greensboro, North Carolina when a car dropped off a man whose physical training and career I admired - Gary Player had arrived for the Greater Greensboro Open. I was too nervous to seek an autograph, and flattered that he lingered to chat while awaiting his wife's arrival. At the time, I was a graduate student at the University of North Carolina and had keys to the Rosenthal Gym, a facility that housed what could best be described as a pitiful strength-training room. The keys ensured I would make a proper fool of myself: I invited Mr. Player to use the facility for the week.

"I don't lift weights during a tournament," he replied, *"but you'll see me jogging around the course this evening."*

It was not what I expected. I assumed that he maintained his strength year-round, despite a hectic schedule. At the same time, I was relieved he rejected the offer: It would have required some fancy footwork.

Gary Player, the gentleman golfer, was everything I expected.

Everything that moves creates friction and that includes swinging a golf club. Friction from the air, from striking the ground and from an unsuspected source – the body - slows movement. Tiny filaments within working muscles slide across each other to create friction during contraction, a phenomenon Arthur Jones called *internal muscle friction*. Friction from this source is heightened by the presence of body fat, which slows speed of movement and explains why all athletes should strive to improve their body composition (muscle-to-fat ratio). Golfers are no exception.

Over-fat golfers (in regard to body composition, not weight) are common at every level of play. It is painful to watch the players of my era - now Champions Tour professionals - who have neglected their bodies to the point that they are no longer effective. To their credit, golf was not considered an *athletic* endeavor in their day, fitness training was not in vogue and many carved out a successful career despite miserable physical status. The aging process, unfortunately, magnifies the misery, and exceptions seem few and far between.

And it comes as no surprise that a small number of current PGA and LPGA professionals do *nothing* in the way of exercise – which leads to a conclusion that provides ammunition when the topic surfaces: *Excellent golf can be played without adherence to an exercise regimen.*

As attractive as it may seem, the assertion doesn't change the facts. Better tools honed through proper training will improve the golf of any player.

Less Body Fat = Less Friction = Greater Speed

Protection from Injury

Every competition, every movement, hosts a contest within – the body's structural integrity *versus* the force to which it is exposed. Injury occurs when external forces exceed the body's tolerance. The instant your body or joint system collides with the high or repetitive forces of movement, superior levels of flexibility, cardiovascular condition, body-fat and skill have little say in the prevention of injury. The key is to develop and maintain an elevated structural integrity via muscle strength. If a golf muscle that is one hundred units strong is exposed to a force of one hundred and one units, something breaks. It also follows, if you double the strength of that same muscle through exercise, a force of two hundred units can be absorbed without a negative outcome. It's a numbers game: The higher the numbers on the side of structural integrity, the less the chance of injury.

Strength provides another advantage. The acquisition of skill in golf requires constant repetition, which takes a physical toll over time. Muscle strength and local muscle endurance (the ability to repeat a contraction) are one and the same, despite the efforts of the fitness industry to establish protocols that suggest otherwise. If the strength of a shoulder muscle is increased by 25 percent through training, its endurance will increase to the same degree. Hitting a few hundred golf balls on the driving range produces fatigue, and reduces the ability of a muscle to produce and withstand force.

Injury caused by repetition can be avoided by conditioning muscles to better handle their demands – through proper strength training.

Can you be too strong for golf?

Judging from the role strength plays in protecting an athlete from injury, the answer is a resounding, "*No.*"

The final two potential benefits of exercise – *body composition and protection from injury* – are by-products of training the other benefits, and generally not considered major reason(s) to adopt a supplemental program of exercise for golf. But the first three are: Golfers will address their strength, flexibility and cardiovascular deficiencies, knowing that progress with *The Big Three* will have a greater impact on performance.

They are correct.

Hole #4 examines the results of training *The Big Three* as supplemental to golf, and will help establish an efficient strategy.

Hole #4: 447 Yards, Par 4

A STRATEGY

Golf + Flexibility

Many tour professionals have adopted stretching as an integral part of their preparation for golf, and the public followed suit: *"If it's good enough for them, it's good enough for us."* Yet, belief in the value of flexibility and its advertized claims has been recently challenged by research:

- Stretching "warms up" muscles.
- Stretching helps prevent injury.
- Stretching helps you recover more quickly from injury.
- Stretching increases flexibility.
- Stretching makes you stronger.

Stretching as a Warm-Up to Prevent or Recover from Injury

Many golfers stretch before play or practice in the belief that it provides a *warm up*. Not so. "Body heat," according to research scientist and writer, Paul Ingraham, "is generated by metabolic activity, particularly muscle contractions."[1] Stretching does not directly involve muscle contraction. The only heat generated by stretching occurs indirectly in the antagonist muscle (the muscle that opposes the one being stretched) which passively contracts to control movement. Ingraham compares the use of stretching as a warm up to "trying to cook a steak by pulling on it," and suggests that "the best way to warm up is to start doing a kinder, gentler version of the activity you have in mind: walk before you run." To add, stretching a muscle before it is warm may lead to injury, which is why many professionals warm up *before* play by performing exercises that *contract* muscles - cardiovascular or light-strength activity - and stretch *after* golf. Research concurs.

A study in the *Clinical Journal of Sports Medicine*, 1999 examined the use of stretching to prevent injury and concluded that *"stretching before exercising does not reduce the risk of injury."*[2] A group of Australian scientists conducted a review of literature examining the effect of pre- and post-exercise stretching on injury prevention and concluded that the effect was minimal to non-existent.[3] Research conducted at the University of Hawaii by David Lally, PhD. found that marathon runners who stretched regularly were at a 33 percent higher risk of injury than runners who did not stretch at all.[4]

And more: Stretching does *not* reduce muscle soreness. Muscle contraction attracts blood flow, and blood is the body's most effective natural healer. Because stretching does *not* involve contraction, it does *not* assist recovery from injury (in this case, the onset of muscle soreness) any more than not stretching at all, a fact confirmed by Australian research: *"Stretching before or after exercising does not confer protection from muscle soreness."*[5]

Stretching to Increase Flexibility

Muscles have a limited range over which they can stretch, a range dictated by joint configuration, and ultimately, by genetics. Just as a rubber band stretched too often loses elasticity, frequent attempts to stretch a muscle beyond its normal limits can gradually weaken tendons and ligaments, a potentially dangerous situation. In a general sense - and though initial gains are possible - stretching should be performed to *maintain* a comfortable range of motion, perhaps the one you have.

Stretching to Increase Strength

Flexibility has no direct relationship to strength. During the stretching process, the antagonist muscle (the one that, by position, opposes the stretch) contracts, but the contraction is passive. If the PNF (Proprioceptive Neuromuscular Facilitation) method of assisted stretching is used, the *active push* against the manual resistance provided by a stretch assistant is a poor stimulus for strength gain, and unintended for that purpose.

A study presented at the 2006 meeting of the American College of Sports Medicine demonstrated that stretching *before* exercise may diminish muscle output. The study examined the effect of stretching the hamstring muscles of the upper thigh before performing a one-repetition maximum test of knee flexion (leg curl). The study compared the effect of one, two, three, four, five and six, 30-second stretches before the test. One 30-second stretch reduced the one-repetition maximum strength by 5.4 percent in eighteen subjects, while six 30-second stretches reduced it by 12.4 percent. This led author, John Little to conclude: "*...since a golfer wants to be stronger and less susceptible to injury, stretching is not something that any rational golfer should engage in.*"[6]

His inference ignores an important point. While the physiological benefits of stretching may be limited, the psychological benefits are not. Stretching can trigger a sensation that you are *ready to go*.

Notes:

Stretching does not contribute to body-fat reduction or improvement in cardiovascular capacity. Its global importance to golf may be overstated.

Golf + Cardiovascular Conditioning

Where an aerobic component is required in golf - walking hilly terrain, for example – an improved cardiovascular capacity speaks for itself. It may also have a positive indirect effect on skill. The efficient delivery of oxygen to the working muscles brought about by progressive aerobic exercise makes you feel physically fit and diminishes fatigue during the final holes of play.

Spending hours on the practice range or playing extra holes leads to sore hands, a reduced focus and the emergence of a *tired* swing – all of which can feed your nervous system erroneous signals. The performance of cardiovascular activity – on a global scale, and not overdone – produces a slight increase in strength and a more efficient delivery of oxygen to the muscles, which increases your ability to repeat a swing or skill.

Too much aerobic activity, however, can lead to strength loss.

I once believed that running was all I needed to create and maintain lower-body strength for golf, and ran twenty-five thousand miles in fifteen years as proof. All the while, I trained my upper-body by lifting weights. When my legs were finally introduced to quality gym equipment, my running went through the roof and put things into perspective: Aerobic activity can make an initial contribution to strength, but will not open the door to your ultimate potential.

The intensity of an aerobic session may be high, but the intensity at the local muscle level is often not. When muscles are taken to exhaustion by aerobic training, the stimulus for strength gain is present but conditions are less than ideal. Strength gain is best accomplished when muscle fatigue occurs between 60-90 seconds – not 60-90 minutes. Therefore, my reaction to a performance of five hundred push-ups remains: *"Congratulations! Now, find a way to make it harder."*

Another point: Cardiovascular training - in any form, and well executed - promotes flexibility loss, because muscles work through a mid-range of motion. They rarely reach positions of full contraction or extension, and lose their ability to stretch over time. If aerobic training is your sole exercise choice to supplement golf, you *must* add a stretching regimen or your swing *will* change.

And, ponder this: *How aerobic is the golf you play?*

Notes:

Aerobic activity reduces body fat, but the process is not as efficient or effective as other forms of exercise. Most trainees believe that burning calories on a treadmill or bike is the best way to reduce fat. Not so. Cardiovascular exercise of any kind results in *indiscriminate weight loss.* That is, calories are burned from fat, organ *and* muscle tissue, which is why - performed in excess - an athlete can lose muscle and strength, and negatively affect his or her muscle-mass/body-fat ratio.

An increase in cardiovascular ability plays a minor role in protecting an athlete from injury. The minimal strength gain attributed to the initial phase of aerobic activity gives it, at best, a weak pass.

Golf + Strength Training

In the late 1960's, I was intrigued by a photo in the clubhouse at the Pinehurst Country Club (NC) of *Toledo Strongman*, Frank Stranahan performing an overhead press with a heavy barbell on the first tee of the famous #2 Course. The two-time British and twice Canadian Amateur champion was runner-up at the Masters in 1947 (as an amateur) and pioneered physical preparation for golf, mentoring the only man on the PGA Tour to perform resistance exercise during my youth, Gary Player.

Back then, strength training was taboo in many sports, which labeled the antics of Stranahan and Player, *eccentric*. As a teen, I often wondered which out-of-shape professional would win the next tournament. Finally, Tiger Woods silenced the crowd by bulldozing his way through the tour and introducing peers to the value of strength and conditioning. Pressured to keep pace, many jumped aboard.

The greatest fear among golfers – especially those who play for a living - is that strength training disrupts skill. Strong muscles represent change, and change requires time. Most trainees quit before benefits are realized. Those who persist reap the rewards.

Strength equips the body and nervous system with better tools to create a swing, facilitate repeated efforts and enhance career longevity.

With proper training and supervision, the average male can add 3-4 pounds of muscle to his body in one month; the average female, 2-3 pounds of muscle in six weeks - which translates to a 25-30 percent increase in strength in traditional 6-12 week research studies. The typical result, while impressive at first glance, failed to excite Arthur Jones, *"If I ever produced only a 25 percent gain in strength from a 12-week training program,"* he said," *I would probably go insane and kill all the subjects."'* Jones conducted a study at West Point in 1975 (outlined on Hole #13) in which he increased the strength of participating cadets by 58.54 percent in six weeks – a statistic that would improve the performance of any activity.

Properly performed - with little to no rest between efforts - strength training can increase cardiovascular ability to levels that equal or surpass that of traditional training. Why?

- The heart *cannot* distinguish source of demand. When a request is made, it responds by increasing its output, and any exercise can trigger the signal – cycling, swimming, lifting weights, or climbing stairs.
- The greater intensity of strength training (*versus* traditional aerobic exercise) elevates the heart rate to a level that can easily be sustained by minimal rest between efforts.

In my first book, *In Arthur's Shadow,* I wrote an article supporting the belief that muscle strength is the limiting factor in cardiovascular capacity, as follows:

Our ultimate cardiovascular capacity (as our potential for strength) is determined by genetics. A review of oxygen pathways - from absorption in the lungs and transportation through the circulatory system, to consumption by the muscle - can help determine what limits that capacity.

The purpose of the lungs is to saturate blood with oxygen, a function easily met under all conditions. At rest, total saturation is accomplished in the first third of the blood's transit time through the lung's capillaries. During maximal exercise, with the heart rate and blood flow increased dramatically and transit time reduced by 50 percent, the reserve capacity of the lungs can easily meet the demand. At the receiving end, muscles are capable of consuming all of the oxygen in the brief period of time it takes the blood to flow through its capillaries, both at rest and during heavy exercise. Therefore, with the lungs and muscles loading and unloading oxygen at near 100 percent efficiency neither appears to be a limiting factor.

The same, however, cannot be said of the circulatory system. Many physiologists believe that the heart itself is the limiting factor, reasoning that if the heart could pump more blood, the body would consume more oxygen. Accordingly, the role of cardiovascular exercise should be to increase the effectiveness of the heart's ability to pump blood. Others claim that the heart can only pump the amount of blood returning to it, and that the peripheral blood vessels restrict the blood's return by resisting every attempt the heart makes to increase blood flow.

When a muscle contracts, internal pressure rises and compresses the blood vessels within, restricting flow. Research demonstrates that such restriction begins with a voluntary contraction of as little as 20 percent and increases proportionately with the intensity of effort. At 50-60 percent (of a maximum contraction), no blood flow is present - and no oxygen delivered or consumed. The system shuts down.

There are only two ways to decrease muscle-contraction intensity during activity:

- *Increase the skill of the individual performing the movement, thereby diminishing the quantity of unnecessary contraction.*
- *Increase the strength of the muscles involved so that each contraction requires a smaller percentage of the available muscle mass.*

Skill is highly specific and requires time to develop, while strength is universal and acquired more efficiently. A distance runner could become a distance swimmer by learning efficient swimming technique. He could improve at both by becoming stronger.

Therefore, in the same way genetic factors dictate our ultimate level of strength, so muscle strength limits our ultimate cardiovascular capacity.[8]

Notes:

Properly performed, progressive resistance exercise goes a long way to protect the body from injury and reduce body fat. Strength training produces a *double reducing effect*: It burns calories *during* exercise (as known), and *after* exercise due to the body's increase in muscle mass.[9] The net effect is greater than that produced by the use of traditional cardiovascular exercise.

Below is a summary of the effect of supplemental exercise options on trainable performance factors.

Summary: Figure 1

The Effect of Supplemental Exercise on Trainable Performance Factors			
	Trainable Performance Factors		
	Skill	**Strength**	**Cardiovascular**
Supplemental Exercise ↓			
Flexibility (Stretching)	0	0	0
Cardiovascular Conditioning	0	1-2	10
Muscle Strengthening	0	10	8-10
0 = No Effect 10 = Full Effect			

The numbers represent opinion, but the facts are clear … and the choice, yours.

References

1. Paul Ingraham, "Quite a Stretch," June (2015). http://www.painscience.com/articles/stretching.php
2. Ian Shrier, "Stretching Before Exercise Does Not Reduce the Risk of Local Muscle Injury: A Critical Review of the Clinical and Basic Science Literature," *Clinical Journal of Sports Medicine* 9 (1999), 221.

3. R.D. Herbert and M. Gabriel, "Effects of Stretching Before and After Exercise on Muscle Soreness and Risk of Injury: Systematic Review," *British Medical Journal* 325 (2002), 468. http://www.ncbi.nlm.nih.gov/pmc/articles/PMC1123979/

4. David Lally, "New Study Links Stretching with Higher Injury Rates," *Running Research News* 10, (1994), 5.

5. R.D. Herbert and M. Gabriel, "Effects of Stretching Before and After Exercise on Muscle Soreness and Risk of Injury: Systematic Review," *British Medical Journal* 325 (2002), 468. http://www.ncbi.nlm.nih.gov/pmc/articles/PMC1123979/

6. John Little, *The Max Golf Workout* (New York: Skyhorse Publishing, 2008), 99.

7. Arthur Jones, "My First Half Century in the Iron Game," Ironman, March (1996), 135.

8. Gary Bannister, *In Arthur's Shadow* (Carmel, IN: Cork Hill Press, 2005), 73.

9. Ellington Darden, *The Nautilus Diet* (Boston, MA: Little, Brown and Company, 1987), 13.

Hole #5: 158 Yards, Par 3

STRENGTH TRAINING PRINCIPLES

1963

Six days before the New Year, my brother and I received a beginner's set of weights from Sears®: one barbell, two dumbbells, several weight-plates, six adjustable red collars and a matching wrench. The 110-pound package came with instructions that encouraged consumers not to die in the process. That summer, we entered the caddy program at the local club where our pre-dawn huddles in the shack adjacent to the tenth tee opened the door to golf on Mondays. When school began, I joined my brother on the high-school cross-country team, which triggered a life-long commitment to aerobic fitness. And finally, within months of receiving the weight-set, an instruction manual from Weider of Canada arrived with illustrated charts and promotional pamphlets.

I vowed to become a fit golfer.

The Weider publication - *The Muscle Building Courses of the Champions* - was laden with tips from the *Master Blaster*, the *Trainer of Champions* himself, Joe Weider – advice that remains in use today:

- Perform multiple sets of each exercise.
- Use low-repetition sets to increase muscle strength; high-repetition sets for muscle endurance.
- Perform fast-paced, explosive repetitions to develop power.
- Perform more exercise as you advance – more days, more sessions per day - up to twenty hours per week.

I followed his advice for approximately eight years, with one exception: I reserved *twenty hours per week* for golf.

1971

The early months of 1971 were equally exciting. My exercise physiology professor at McMaster University, Dr. Digby Sale, called me to his office months before graduation to share what he had received by mail. His packet contained information and glossy photos of a new product called a *thinking man's barbell*, a *Nautilus Time Machine*. Dr. Sale's rare enthusiasm was off the charts. Months later, he proudly escorted me to a small room in the basement of the physical education complex to unveil the school's first Nautilus plate-loaded Pullover machine.

The equipment, I would learn, was based on design features hitherto unknown; but the new company represented more than tools. Nautilus Sports/Medical Industries® had a unique training philosophy, not exclusive to their brand:

- Perform one set of each exercise to muscle failure.
- Work each muscle group no more than twice a week.
- Move slowly and smoothly during each repetition (regardless of the desired training effect).
- Perform 8-12 repetitions for optimal increases in both muscle strength *and* muscle endurance.

The novel ideas were born of Nautilus inventor Arthur Jones, a scientist and logical thinker, who, by trial and error, developed a more efficient and effective muscle-building formula. His blunt method of communication ruffled a few feathers.

1973

I first experienced the practical application of Jones' theory at a Nautilus gym in Danville, Virginia in 1973 when a fellow professor invited me to workout. There was nothing, I thought, that Coach couldn't handle. Coach was wrong. I ended up on the floor after two exercises, and in the bathroom midway through the fourth. The experience was an embarrassment to someone who thought he was in great shape, and was - but it was common. The intensity delivered by the new tools made barbell training feel like child's play, and threw my system into shock. I later learned that, during the first four years at Nautilus headquarters in Lake Helen, Florida (1970-1974), no trainee finished a twelve-exercise circuit under Jones' supervision. That eased the pain, but didn't change the facts.

From that day forward, I subscribed to the new training principles and began to comprehend the underlying concepts. Books by Ellington Darden, PhD., Director of Research for Nautilus, articles by Arthur Jones in *The Athletic Journal* and *Ironman* magazine, and a handful of lectures conducted by the Nautilus inventor heightened my interest and insight. I was not alone.

Nautilus facilities began flooding the country, but not everyone was on board. The *Trainer of Champions* began to dismantle everything associated with the new system by means of an entourage of assorted goons - physicians, physiologists and bodybuilders - and through his publication empire. Arthur Jones posed a threat.

The back and forth continued for years – Weider *versus* Jones, machines *versus* free-weights, one set *versus* three, high-intensity *versus* volume training. Everyone took a side.

2004

December, 2004 provided a measure of resolution. Two British researchers, Dave Smith and Stewart Bruce-Low of the Department of Sport and Exercise Sciences at the University of Liverpool, published an article in the *Journal of the American Society of Exercise Physiologists* titled, "Strength Training Methods and the Work of Arthur Jones."

They first examined three of Jones' books (*Nautilus Training Principles, Bulletin No. 1*, 1970; *Nautilus Training Principles, Bulletin No. 2*, 1971; and *The Lumbar Spine*, 1988) and more than one hundred published articles to extract his core ideas and compare their effectiveness to the widely-accepted ideas of the day, using scientific research and analysis.

Number of Sets

The duo reviewed forty-one studies that compared the results produced by single versus multiple sets and found that many references cited in books and articles were opinions, not actual studies backed by scientific evidence. They concluded, "...*the great majority of well-controlled, peer-reviewed studies support Jones' contention that one set to failure is all that is necessary to stimulate optimal increases in muscular size and strength.*"[1]

Frequency

The pair examined ten studies related to exercise frequency and found that optimal outcomes resulted from training each muscle twice a week, as Jones suggested.

More time for golf.

Speed of Movement

Smith and Bruce-Low examined twenty studies that explored speed of movement during exercise and arrived at two outcomes: *One*, that slow training was superior to explosive training (for strength and power); and *Two*, that there was no *significant* difference between slow and fast speeds. In four studies, they identified and exposed the serious risk of injury from *explosive* training. "*It appears that Jones' recommendation,*" they concluded, "*that slow, controlled weight training is all that is necessary to enhance both muscular strength and power is correct.*"[2]

Number of Repetitions

The research duo reviewed eight studies related to repetition range – the number of repetitions required to produce best results. The studies revealed that low-to-moderate repetition schemes produced optimal results *as well as* proportionate increases in strength and muscular endurance. Low-repetition schemes did *not* produce better strength gains, but demonstrated a greater inherent danger to joint and connective tissue. High-repetition schemes were of *no* value to the production of muscle endurance. A range of eight to twelve (8-12) repetitions was declared, "...*effective and prudent.*"

More time for golf.

Conclusion

The work of Smith and Bruce-Low - the validation of Jones' original training concepts (*The Nautilus System*) – had little impact. Bodybuilders failed to understand the new approach - just as they had failed to understand their own – and rejected the concept of *less* exercise and the use of machines in general.

The field of exercise has recently taken the debate a step beyond by rejecting single-station machines that isolate muscles on the grounds that isolation is *non-functional*. The current bashing leads to the heart and soul of this publication.

Arthur Jones called it his way, *"An open mind is not the same as an empty head."*

Strength Training Principles

Throughout my association with golf-exercise programs, I have distributed literature to educate clients, and wish to clarify:

General Strength Training Principles for Golf (below) is *not* an attempt to commercialize or modify the original concepts of strength training to suit a golfing population. Strength training principles have universal application – to swimming, tennis, football, rehabilitation, wrestling, etc. Golfers are special people, but they do *not* require special strength training principles, as some would have you believe. The concepts that follow are original to Nautilus, tried and proven, and in possession of every client I have trained *for golf.*

Work hard, and enjoy the time you save.

General Strength Training Principles for Golf

Intensity

1. The higher the intensity during exercise, the greater the chance of improving strength.

2. Gradually increase intensity (*as a short-term goal*) until each exercise is continued to a point of momentary muscle fatigue (*a long-term goal*).

3. Keep rest to a minimum between exercises to increase overall workout intensity.

4. For best results: push yourself, train with a partner, or have your workouts supervised.

Form

1. When using exercise machines, adjust the seat height or position of your body to align your joint system with the rotational axis of the machine. Use all seat belts provided.

2. Perform each exercise with a slow speed of movement (*2-3 seconds to lift/4-5 seconds to lower*) through a complete range of motion. Use a speed that allows you to feel the muscle *lift* the weight throughout. Avoid fast or jerky movements.

3. Relax all body parts not involved in the exercise. Exhale during the lifting phase, recover during the lowering phase. Avoid making faces, holding your breath or grasping machine handles tightly during your efforts.

4. Exercise in strict form until fatigue sets in; then, cheat minimally for 1-2 final repetitions.

5. On most exercises, lift the weight to a contracted position and pause briefly (*1-2 seconds*). Exceptions include movements that push away from your body's center (*leg, chest and shoulder presses; squats and dips*) where a locking limb or brief pause provides a rest.

Progression

1. Attempt to increase weight or repetitions during every workout. If you cannot complete eight repetitions in good form, the weight is too heavy; if you complete twelve or more repetitions in good form, increase the weight by approximately five percent.

2. If twelve repetitions are surpassed during exercise (*because the selected weight is too light*), continue until movement is no longer possible. Then, adjust the weight for the next session.

3. Keep training records and set daily, weekly and long-term goals.
4. Avoid one-repetition maximum lifts. Your goal is to increase, not demonstrate, strength.

Other

1. Select exercises that provide the greatest range of motion for the major muscle groups (*or those involved in your sport*). In general, the larger the muscle mass involved, the greater the value of the exercise.
2. Perform 4-6 lower-body exercises and 6-8 upper-body exercises – a total of twelve.
3. Work large muscles first, small ones last (*in order: hips, legs, torso, arms, abdomen, others*).
4. Keep workouts brief (*20-25 minutes on machines*), and allow 48-72 hours between sessions.
5. Vary workouts (*sequence, emphasis and equipment*) to keep motivated.
6. Warm-up before (*approximately five minutes*) and cool-down after vigorous strength training. In general, perform progressive-resistance exercise before cardiovascular exercise.
7. Advanced trainees require *less* exercise than beginners because of the body's limited recovery capacity – a capacity that diminishes as strength increases.

Hole #6 examines the difference(s) between the basic principles of skill training and strength training.

References

1. Dave Smith and Stewart Bruce-Low, "Strength Training Methods and the Work of Arthur Jones," *Journal of the American Society of Exercise Physiologists* 7, no. 6 (2004).
2. Dave Smith and Stewart Bruce-Low, "Strength Training Methods and the Work of Arthur Jones," *Journal of the American Society of Exercise Physiologists* 7, no. 6 (2004).

Hole #6: 405 Yards, Par 4

SKILL TRAINING
VS
STRENGTH TRAINING

I stood on the back of the third green at Lookout Point as I had hundreds of times, with one glaring difference: I had no clubs. The foursome I followed that day had, so far, earned a yawn - a yawn that was interrupted by a commotion on the adjacent seventh, a lengthy par five. To my right, like a bolt of lightning, I caught glimpse of a stout man snatch a club from the Sunday bag he carried and rifle a shot down the middle of the fairway – all *before* the bag hit the ground.

Lookout hosted the Ontario Pro-Pro competition that spring. I regret not watching Moe Norman play a complete round of golf at my home course.

I had witnessed the legend during an exhibition at the Hamilton Golf Club in Ancaster, Ontario, when my eyesight was perfect. He hit hundreds of balls in rapid succession: *Not one* curved left, *not one* curved right.

In a December, 1995 *Golf Digest* article, the author compared Norman's ability to mechanically repeat the golf swing to that of *Iron Byron*, a machine named after Byron Nelson, and considered the gold standard of club and ball testing.

It's hard to believe that anyone could perfect a skill that so playfully eludes everyone who has ever taken up the challenge - with one exception. The only other acknowledged pure ball-striker in the history of the game was Ben Hogan. And while I witnessed 60-year-old Sam Snead win the PGA

Championship for club professionals at Pinehurst, NC in the early 1970's, I never had the opportunity to view his contemporary, Mr. Hogan – a second regret.

A high level of skill in golf is elusive. Furthermore, many believe that such a level - achieved through practice - is jeopardized the moment they embark on a strength training program. Naturally, such naysayers are attracted to programs that offer a more direct, but gentle approach. Don't be fooled.

The blend of strength training and skill training inherent in today's golf performance programs is *not* the ticket to the Promised Land:

> *Movement and performance depend on two major factors: muscle strength and skill. The result of muscle contraction (the strength system) is the performance of a skill controlled by the central nervous system (the skill system). Contributions by inherited abilities affect the quality of the final product.*

> *(Nautilus inventor) Jones believed that training to improve skill and training to improve strength must remain apart. Skill training is specific, must precisely mimic the activity or skill one is trying to improve with no alteration of any factor that could influence the practice or performance of the skill, including a change of resistance. Effective skill training requires no resistance other than that of the implement used in the performance of the skill (tennis racquet, golf club, shot put, etc.). In addition, the intensity of skill training must prevent a high level of fatigue, which could negatively affect the quality of performance (a fresh versus fatigued effort).*

> *Strength training on the other hand, is general in its application. A strong triceps will help any movement that involves triceps. In addition, best results from strength training require what Jones called 'outright hard work' – the use of maximum overload, intensity and fatigue to stimulate change.[1]*

The differences between training for skill and training for strength are clear. Effective skill acquisition requires no resistance, adherence to specificity, a low-to-moderate level of effort (unless intense efforts are required of the skill) and brief, frequent training sessions. Effective strength training, on the other hand, requires a maximum overload (for 8-12 repetitions), no specificity, a high level of intensity and brief, infrequent training sessions. A comparison is illustrated below:

Training Parameter	Skill	Strength
Overload (Resistance)	Zero	Maximum
Intensity	Low-Moderate	High
Duration	Brief	Brief
Frequency	Frequent	Infrequent
Application to Sport	Specific	General

The only parameter common to both skill training and strength training is the recommended brevity of workouts. In the case of skill, slugging hundreds of balls on the driving range to perfect a swing can lead to physical and mental fatigue. Furthermore, practicing a skill in a fatigued state leads to errors that may require future attention. Moe Norman, to be clear, hit so quickly that his 500-ball practice sessions remained brief by today's standards.

In 1963, at a driving range in Toronto, Moe Norman hit 1,540 consecutive golf balls with a driver, taking a five minute break each hour.

Despite soreness and bleeding, Moe was not concerned that fatigue would affect a skill that was so ingrained.

Apparently, it did not.

From a strength perspective, workout intensity and duration are mutually exclusive - if you have one you *cannot* have the other. If your workout is as intense as it must be to stimulate change, it will not last long; if it is long in duration, it can't be hard. That logic applies to every physical endeavor, including those of today's more-is-better advocates. *Strength gain requires intensity, and intensity demands brevity –* something many golf professionals have yet to grasp.

Despite the obvious differences between skill and strength training, some genius decided to combine the two to produce a hybrid form of exercise called *functional training*, strength training with a higher calling. The hybrid was then applied to sports, and became known as *sport-specific training*. The concept caught on. Global organizations such as the National Academy of Sports Medicine (NASM) launched a massive campaign to certify trainers in the new form of exercise. All the while, instructors began to combine training modalities to reach a broader audience: Pilates merged with Yoga, dance with core training, vibration technology with traditional exercise and - last but not least - skill training with strength training.

One thing was clear: No one did their homework; and worse, no one cared about doing homework.

The motivation for change was, for the most part, economic. Golfers reluctant to perform traditional strength training needed a brighter lure. Testimonials from those who had tried the old and failed, as well as whispers from the past, cast aside the observations of a man who trained thousands of subjects – some, the best athletes on the planet:

"...in the meantime, it has been clearly and repeatedly demonstrated hundreds of times, with no single exception I ever heard of and no exception I would believe unless I saw it myself, that proper strength training will markedly improve the performance of any athlete in any sport."[2]

Despite a life-long search for truth, Arthur Jones knew that trainees would not embrace his approach. Proper strength training is hard work, and the average person is *not willing* to perform hard work. A gentler something would surely have greater appeal – especially if it was perceived as *functional*, or looked *like golf*.

During a golf exhibition in Orlando, Florida, Moe Norman stopped for a moment to address the crowd. *"I want to show you how the pros like to hit,"* he uttered. *"They like to draw the ball from right to left."* He struck a seven-iron that featured a gentle draw. *"Now,"* he continued, *"they think that's pretty. I think it stinks. You want to see pure? Watch that flag."* He pointed to a target about 160 yards away and hit approximately twenty-five shots at a three-to-four second interval. Ball after ball landed at the foot of the flagstick, as if someone had tipped an overhead bucket. There wasn't a shut jaw in the crowd. When *Pipeline* Moe ceased fire, he said in a matter of fact tone, *"Now that's pure."*

The holes that follow reveal exactly what the pros think is *pretty* as far as golf conditioning is concerned: At the same time, they clearly demonstrate what is *pure*. A special training program for golf - when you know the facts – is neither necessary nor *functional*, and may have best been defined well in advance of its arrival:

"Remember – you can have an elephant's body, an elephant's head, four elephant's feet, and all of the other required parts, but you still won't have an elephant if all of the required parts are not fitted together properly."[3]

In the case of golf, the parts don't fit.

References

1. Gary Bannister, *If You Like Exercise … Chances Are You're Doing It Wrong* (Bloomington, IN: iUniverse, 2013), 128.
2. Arthur Jones, "The Relationship of Strength to Functional Ability in Sports." In *Total Fitness: The Nautilus Way*, edited by James A. Peterson (New York: Leisure Press, 1978), 163.
3. Arthur Jones, *Nautilus Training Principles, Bulletin No. 2* (Self published, 1971), 102.

Hole #7: 526 Yards, Par 5

FUNCTIONAL TRAINING

In an endless quest for something new, the field of exercise has created a dandy. Traditional strength training - performed with free-weights or machines - has been displaced by what experts claim is a method more apt to improve the performance of day-to-day activities: Its catchy name, *functional training.*

Despite its popularity and growth, advocates can barely agree on a definition. According to Paul Chek in *Movement That Matters*, functional training is *"any type of exercise that relates directly to the activities you perform in your daily life ... in other words, functional training is reality-based: Your body mimics everyday movements that you already perform, but want to perform better."*[1] He calls it *"action-specific, movement-specific or sports-specific training,"* where it extends to the game of golf.

Nor is there agreement on its proper application. Some experts advocate the duplication of everyday activities *without* the use of added resistance (the performance of a squat with no resistance other than body-weight, for example, is the best way to help a person bend to pick something off the floor). Others believe that all movements should be duplicated *with* added resistance. *With* or *without* represents the least of their concerns.

Let's identify the basic premises of functional training, according to those in-the-know:

The body works as a whole and must be trained as such - using movement patterns that incorporate muscle integration and multi-joint exercise. Muscle isolation in daily activities and sports, they claim, is rare and should remain absent from exercise, rehabilitation and strength assessment.

Train the movement, not the muscle. Exercise should focus on skill and movement patterns, challenge the nervous system without disrupting the motor-learning process (due to complexity or intensity), and address the needs of the trainee (determined by a general movement screen).

Exercise should occur in an unstable environment to activate the body's static-stabilizer and postural systems. The support of benches (with free-weights) or seats (with machines) during traditional training promotes the pathological loading of ligaments and joint instability by not allowing the body to learn its own balance and stability. This learning process, according to functional advocates, can be enhanced by practicing high-skill movements and full-body exercises using tools that challenge balance - Swiss balls, balance boards and vibration platforms. *"Stability,"* they say, *"must always precede force generation."*

Exercise should promote, encourage or replicate primal movement patterns - general innate motor abilities that do not require special skill (twisting, pulling, pushing, lunging, bending and squatting). The common inability to efficiently perform primal patterns at a subconscious level should be identified by a movement assessment, and addressed by the application of an appropriate *functional* remedy.

Transfer exists between skills or activities. Repetition of a movement *similar to* the activity you are trying to improve has a positive effect on the performance of the target activity. And more: The quality of one action extends to other actions. For example, the *explosive* nature of the clean-and-jerk (a power-lifting staple) makes athletes more *explosive* during play.

Functional training can improve common abilities that support and underlie skills – abilities such as balance, hand/eye coordination and agility.

Not everyone agrees with functional experts, let alone the concept of experts.

When asked how he acquired his exercise expertise, Arthur Jones replied, *"There are no experts in any field. There are some people arrogant enough to call themselves experts and many people dumb enough to believe them. I quit school in grade four. I'm not an expert in anything."*[2]

Let's view the same premises from the other side of the coin.

The body works, and must be trained, as a whole.

Dr. Greg Bradley-Popovich (DPT, MSEP, MS, CSCS, CEI), Director of Clinical Research, NW Spine Management, Rehabilitation and Sports Conditioning, Portland, Oregon, challenges the exclusive use of multi-joint exercises to strengthen movement patterns and correct functional deficiencies, as follows:

> *Within a rehabilitative context, functional training may be described as training that mimics elements of the complex movements of daily living. Although I am not opposed to all forms of functional training and believe select exercises can be successfully implemented when used judiciously, the manner in which functional training is commonly implemented, in my view, is flawed. Most commonly, functional training movements are compound (i.e., multi-joint) motions with the underlying logic being that most real-life movements are in fact compound. Herein lies the problem: if only complex motions are used to overload a movement pattern, then the best conditioned muscles in the kinetic chain can accept the brunt of the work. In other words, use of compound movements may do nothing at all to stimulate a weak muscle in the chain because other muscles are permitted to substitute. As the compensating muscles grow stronger, the strength disparity between the substituting muscles and the weakened muscle(s) may grow greater. Such imbalances may lead to increased biomechanical stress (i.e., wear and tear).*

> *While it is true that a chain is only as strong as its weakest link, this is true of only relatively simple movements. In contrast, gross movements of multiple-body segments may be accomplished by a number of subtly different means—and therefore by a number of different muscles. A prime example of how muscles can compensate is the relationship of the muscles involved in trunk extension: paraspinal lumbar muscles, gluteals, and hamstrings. In patients with chronic low back pain, isolated paraspinal muscle strength is typically diminished. But, any attempt to overload the low back muscles through a supposedly functional task such as lifting weighted boxes may be nullified by compensatory involvement of the hamstrings and gluteals with no meaningful exercise delivered*

to the low back. And, the small muscles of the low back are the only muscles in a position to finely control motion of individual vertebral segments. Natural muscle synergies such as the cooperative efforts of the aforementioned muscles of truncal extension are truly synergistic only if each contributing muscle pulls its own weight, so to speak.

The lesson to be learned from the number of aberrant muscle substitution pathways is that weak links need to be identified early through isolated analysis and trained in an isolated fashion. Efforts to overload complex movements while ignoring inherent weak links are most often misdirected.[3]

The movement screen in common use with functional programs is designed to identify deficiencies without *isolating* muscles, in part because isolation within the system is taboo. The evaluation involves, among other tests, performance of an *overhead squat* - extending a non-weighted stick above your head while lowering to a full-squat position in order to *identify* functional weakness. Once a weakness is detected, its manner of correction is, according to Dr. Bradley-Popovich, flawed. The exclusive use of multi-joint exercises and whole-body participation to correct a specific developmental weakness is akin to asking your dentist to drill all of your teeth when the problem is located in one.

To add, the exclusive use of multi-joint exercises is a step backwards in regard to strength acquisition. More on that later ...

Train the movement, not the muscle.

Functional advocates believe that *the body knows nothing of muscles, only of movement,* and that training should focus on movement, rather than on the muscles that produce movement. When I first heard that, several things sprung to mind:

- How do you *train* movement? Movement training is skill training, a process that belongs (in this case) in the hands of golf professionals. And ...
- If the body knows *nothing of muscles,* how will it know *movement?* Without muscle contraction there is no movement.

59

Functional exercises, claim the experts, score high on a scale of motor complexity (require greater skill than traditional training), which increases the likelihood of establishing a qualitative physical impression on the nervous system, but for this. The qualitative impression on the nervous system belongs to a skill foreign to the one you are trying to improve.

It gets worse. *"The integration of full-body participation,"* claims Paul Chek, *"is best accomplished by performing exercise on a Swiss ball."*

How does Swiss-ball training improve physical impressions on nerve tissue when you consider the specific nature of an impression relative to each unique task? Being good at Swiss-ball exercise A, for example, does not guarantee success at Swiss-ball exercise B, or at non-Swiss-ball tasks. Skill patterns are unique, and do *not* transfer to other tasks.

Functional experts are correct on one point. If a single-joint exercise is performed to strengthen a muscle (which I've yet to see in performance training), then *"adequate time must be spent training the muscle to contribute to a functional movement pattern."*[4]

As true as it is, the statement implies that adequate time would *not* be necessary, if strength training had been combined with skill training in the first place.

Who's kidding who? The only way the body learns how to use its strength to best advantage is through skill training alone.

Training skill patterns against resistance compromises both skill and strength components, and is based on three false premises:

1. That *specificity* in skill training does not exist.
2. That skill *transfer* occurs automatically when you practice an activity that is similar to - but not exact to - the original skill.
3. That a muscle can reach its strength potential through the exclusive use of multi-joint exercises.

One and two were negated by motor learning research fifty years ago. The third may reflect current trends, but is utterly false.

Exercise should occur in an unstable environment.

Functional advocates continually reference the importance of the body's static stabilizer or postural system - a system that doesn't exist. Why? Every muscle in the body experiences the act of stabilization at one time or another, independent of a *system*.

Muscles require two attachment points to contract: They attach from *somewhere* (origin) and go to *somewhere* (insertion). The multi-joint approach to training insists that muscles work freely across both attachments, which render leg-curl machines *useless* - one joint (the knee) is fixed. Yet, functional advocates are blind to the following:

- That movement of some everyday activities occurs at one joint only.
- That leg presses and squats, which engage hip and knee joints simultaneously, are *functional* by definition, yet rarely employed.
- What requires a muscle to act as an antagonist in one task may require it to act as a stabilizer - or agonist - in another.
- That the performance of highly unstable exercises on a *balance* tool (Swiss-ball, balance board, or other apparatus) does *not* improve stability and balance in another activity. How can practicing instability in one task *increase* stability in another? The only weakness improved by the use of a balance tool is the skill itself - proper performance on the apparatus.

Some get it ...

Dr. Michael Fulton, orthopedic representative for MedX Corporation, received a call from a disgruntled niece in Iowa and offered her a position as a physical therapist in his state-of-the-art rehabilitation facility in Daytona Beach, Florida. Things worked well for about a year. One morning, Dr. Fulton walked into the clinic and spotted a collection of colored balls and latex tubing with handles. *"First thing,"* he said, *"I pulled out my penknife."* He punctured the balls and cut the tubing, which prompted his niece to resign, claiming she could not work with people who were not her kind. The doctor verified his stance to me by phone, *"We're all homo sapiens, aren't we?"*

A word about stability: The body likes to know where it is - and where it's supposed to be - when we learn skills, and does so through a hierarchy (in order):

1. The body and mind establish proper posture. The head, neck, trunk, spine and other body segments coordinate with foot placement to produce an ideal base of support, if not already established.
2. Large muscle groups near the center of the body (hips, thighs, upper back and chest) contract to keep the body balanced relative to the action being performed.
3. Small muscle groups in the peripheral areas contract and work with the basic postural and motor components.

In essence, basic (innate) motor skills are taken care of *prior to* the execution of a task. Regardless of speed of movement, the process remains constant - large muscles contract first, followed by small - to produce an orderly, efficient movement pattern as determined through the acquired skills.

The same applies to the execution of an exercise. The body stabilizes itself - without conscious effort or training - *before* generating force, which exposes other concepts ignored by functional experts:

- Stability and large-to-small muscle integration occurs during *all* exercise - is *not* limited to functional exercise - and should not be considered exclusive to functional improvement.
- The stability requirements of each sport skill, everyday activity and *functional* exercise are unique. Consequently, functional training exercise *cannot* enhance stability or balance in an unlike task any better than traditional exercise.

Exercise should focus on primal movement patterns.

Primal patterns - as defined in *Movement That Matters* - are natural, *innate* movement patterns based on ability. The author (Paul Chek) believes that the average person cannot successfully perform primal patterns (squatting, pushing or pulling) because he or she lacks skill. He then introduces movement patterns in the form of exercises that correct the deficient skills. I thought I'd heard it all.

Innate means inborn, genetic, not subject to change. Why spend time and energy on something that cannot be improved? Besides, the inability to complete a primal movement pattern may be due to a genetic problem, an injury that affects the ability to perform or a de-conditioned body, in which case a traditional fitness program would prepare the body to better perform the task. *Lack of use* is more likely the cause of performance issues than *deficient motor patterns.*

Transfer exists between activities.

The skill acquired through the practice of an exercise remains unique to that exercise. Practice of a Nautilus-machine chest press, for example, increases skill on that machine only. Practice of a free-weight chest press on a flat bench increases chest-press skill with free weights on that bench. The same with a chest press performed on a Swiss ball - you eventually master the skill required. While none of the skills acquired in one chest-press exercise assist those acquired in another, the strength gained in any of the presses may increase performance in the others. Strength is general and transfers from one activity to another; skill is specific and does not.

To illustrate the point, IART founder Brian Johnston suggests attempting an agility drill in frequent use with athletes (to paraphrase):

> *First, hop laterally (side to side) over a small stool, box or object (under 6-8 inches high) for 10-15 repetitions. Now, try the same with your ankles tied together, and note: The lack of space between your feet alters the motor pattern.*
>
> *Next, untie your legs and hop with an uneven rhythm (a hop-hop-pause-hop-hop-hop-pause - or any other arrhythmic combination). Now, tie your ankles and try the same. The alteration of the timing interferes with what was previously practiced as your mind and body strive to maintain a steady rhythm, regardless of the speed of movement. A simple change creates a drastic difference in skill application. Now, consider how removed these lateral hops are to actual athletic events that may require lateral agility in a different environment, with a different stimuli and measure of application. Beyond simple improvement in physical condition, these agility drills have no purpose.[5]*

The transfer of skill assumed by the performance of an activity in the gym that replicates a skill involved in a sport *does not exist*. And that includes the skill(s) of golf. Any attempt to include such *like* activities under the umbrella of exercise is, at best, a waste of time.

Arthur Jones summed it up forty years ago: "*...Specificity in strength training is an outright myth, an utter impossibility ... and it's a good thing that it is impossible, because it has absolutely no value in the way of increasing strength; and ... anything approaching specificity is even worse, because it will do little or nothing to increase strength but it will hurt your skills.*"[6]

Abilities can be improved by functional training.

Skills are specific. Abilities (such as balance, agility and hand-eye coordination) are underlying genetic traits that support skill performance. Functional experts are convinced that abilities can be improved through practice. They believe that balance sensors activated in the practice of Skill A, for example, improve the balance parameters of Skill B because the same sensors are involved. The idea is creative and logical, but false. The claimed increase in balance on a task is due to an improvement in skill related to that task. When balance forms an integral part of a skill, it improves only in relation to that skill, and does *not* improve balance in a different skill (because of its unique requirements). To repeat, balance - among other abilities - is genetically determined, formed at an early age, not subject to change and does not transfer from one skill to another. If trained as a global concept - by use of a general balance activity that may assist any skill requiring its input – trainees master nothing more than a repertoire of useless skills under the illusion that their balance has improved. Effective training must be tailored to the task: *To improve the balance required to exit a deep sofa, bring in the sofa.*

The same applies to agility and hand-eye coordination.

I marvel at PGA Tour ads that portray the talents of their professionals. "*This guy can dunk a basketball,*" "*This guy was a fearless motocross champion,*" etc. Other than human-interest stories, the ability to play high-level golf is totally unrelated to one's ability to dunk a basketball or ride a motorbike.

Observations

In an endless quest for something new, the sport of golf has introduced a few dandies of its own.

One: The designer of the course at which I caddied, Walter Travis, took up the game of golf at age thirty-five. Within two years, he reached the semifinals of the US Amateur and by then, had adopted the name, *The Old Man*. *"My experiments,"* he explained, *"were confined almost exclusively to driving and iron play generally, the gentle art of putting being left to take care of itself, with the result that for the first two or three years I was quite weak on the putting green."*[7] He eventually refined his putting skills and won the first of three US Amateur Championships in 1900.

In 1904, 43-year-old Travis traveled to Royal St. Georges to compete in the world's oldest amateur event, the British Amateur. In his bag was *"the best putter I have ever used,"* a center-shafted aluminum-head mallet purchased from GE engineer, Arthur Knight of the Mohawk Golf Club, Schenectady, NY in 1902. Within a week of Walter's endorsement of what became known as the *Schenectady putter*, more than one hundred orders were placed with Knight.

During the event in England, Travis sunk nearly every putt he looked at to the chagrin of the British public, and became the first non-Brit to win *their* tournament – a feat not repeated for twenty-two years. The victory ignited a controversy that lasted until 1910 when *"center-shafted, mallet-headed implements"* were banned by The Royal and Ancient Golf Club in St. Andrews, Scotland. The ban was lifted in 1951. For a brief time, everyone scrambled to get their hands on the magic tool, just as they now consider *functional training* the magic tool for golf.

Two: I joined a similar scramble following Moe Norman's exhibition in Orlando, Florida. Several *Natural Golf* instructors invited anyone from the crowd to partake in a brief lesson. I learned two things: It's tough to rotate your shoulders around a dropped jaw; and tougher to replicate a swing with clubs as heavy as baseball bats. The added resistance amounted to learning a new skill. Where was the R & A when I needed them?

Three: My first sports hero, Eddie Feigner, faced what he hoped was his last batter. The pitcher of the famous four-man softball team, *The King and his Court,* had the upper hand - two outs, two strikes on the batter in the bottom of the seventh, and a one-run lead on a nine-man All-Star Team. Feigner heard a cry from the umpire, *"Time."* The opposing coach took the batter aside, *"He likes to throw the last pitch of the game behind his back."* Eddie raised his muscular arm to its apex and swerved it to his backside on the down. Coach was right ... but late. The catcher's mitt made its familiar sound; and the umpire his, *"SteeeRike!"* The All-Star bench and crowd descended on the ump. Feigner sped to a waiting van, ball in hand, and listened as they argued over a pitch he called *The Phantom. "They thought it was too high,"* he chuckled. The facts were clear: Few could see, let alone hit, any pitch of Feigner's - which ultimately created room for discussion; and everyone was caught in the frenzy of a high pitch. No one bothered to check the catcher's mitt. By the time the smoke cleared, *The King* was halfway to the next town.

It's human nature to get caught up in the frenzy of the moment. Whether it's the latest implement or method in golf, or the latest call in sports, we take sides, often without checking credentials. Or we feel obligated to get involved because everyone is. The field of exercise is not immune to such frenzy, and should be approached with a measure of caution:

"If you want to discover something about exercise," said Arthur Jones, *"write down all of your questions, go to a local gym and find the biggest guy there. Ask him every question and record every word he says. Then, take the information home and do the exact opposite. You'll be one step in the right direction."*

Brian Johnston summed it up best:

> *"It is ironic that even after a concept is explained in simple terms, so that a child can understand, that well educated, intelligent people will continue to ignore the facts and the common sense arguments put forth in this critique. They uphold their biases because of politics or ego. They refuse to listen or understand in order to sustain their beliefs, and often to sustain the financial niche they have created for themselves in the marketplace (a niche based on falsehood).*

If the reader considers him or herself a student of science, it is vital that the concept of cause and effect be accepted, rather than coincidence. We must uphold that standard before going off half-cocked to accept what we think might be true, based on casual observation or what 'authorities' tell us. Authorities ... are not always correct, and neither am I, for that matter. We must weigh the evidence relative to what is known and what is fact (and common sense in many instances) and draw our conclusions accordingly."[8]

Why the lengthy discussion on functional training, you ask? It provides the philosophical and practical base for sports performance training, and sport-specific exercise. When its concepts are applied to golf, it makes the 1963 instruction sheet that accompanied my first set of barbells from Sears® look mighty attractive ...

References

1. Paul Chek, *Movement That Matters* (Vista, CA: C.H.E.K. Institute, 1999).
2. Arthur Jones, "20 Questions: Arthur Jones," Playboy (March, 1983), 126.
3. Brian Johnston, *System Analysis* (Sudbury, ON: Bodyworx Publishing, 2001), 142.
4. Paul Chek, *Movement That Matters* (Vista, CA: C.H.E.K. Institute, 1999).
5. Brian Johnston, *System Analysis* (Sudbury, ON: Bodyworx Publishing, 2001), 171.
6. Arthur Jones, "Specificity in Strength Training ... The Facts and Fables," *Athletic Journal*, May (1977).
7. MatthewM, "Walter Travis," *thegolfforum* July (2012), http://www.thegolfforum.com/index.php?/topic/5610-walter-travis/
8. Brian Johnston, *System Analysis* (Sudbury, ON: Bodyworx Publishing, 2001), 177.

Hole #8: 175 Yards, Par 3

FUNCTIONAL TRAINING FOR GOLF

I recently unearthed a series of four-page pamphlets issued by Nautilus Sports/Medical Industries® in reference to physical preparation for sports. Their common thread was an analysis of major muscle groups used in the sport, a selection of exercises to strengthen those muscles, and sample workouts to accomplish the task. I once posted the workouts throughout my facility in Caracas, Venezuela in 1980, and modified the offerings when new equipment arrived.

One thing stood out - the similarity among programs for different purposes. The swimming program, with slight modification, was similar to the baseball and golf programs. And the running proposal was akin to that of tennis - but no one blinked. The use of an established routine was not an attempt to pull wool over anyone's eyes, but rather an effort to share the best information available at the time - and, it made sense. A hamstring is a hamstring, and if it was used in your sport, the Leg Curl machine was on your menu, with one choice - prone or seated?

If you view the big picture, ask a golfer to identify one muscle he or she does *not* use during the swing. Then, ask the same of a tennis player, swimmer or volleyball star. The silence is deafening. Most sports engage the same large muscle groups (with some variation in emphasis), a fact that does not sit well with everyone. The one-shoe-fits-all approach to training was challenged in the 1970's by those who considered themselves - or their sport of choice – *special;* and by those who sought an alternative to *lifting weights.*

Golfers, for one, failed to understand the role of strength in their high-skill sport. They challenged the intensity of traditional exercise routines (*"We're not playing football"*) or blamed their lousy weekend performance on Friday's workout. Foursomes listened, and word spread.

The industry rushed to the rescue with something new – functional exercise for golf – an easier pill to swallow, rationalize and sell. The final product – by now, named *sport-specific* or *performance* training – sprung to the forefront and triggered a massive scramble for prominence. In the end, money, television exposure and a global certification effort prevailed to create the *gold standard* of exercise programs for golf, the Titleist Performance Institute Program, or TPI.

All that glitters is not gold.

From start to finish, TPI is nothing more than functional training applied to golf with all the trappings of an empire: a thorough physical analysis to determine the needs of the client, the selection of corrective measures to address deficiencies, the execution of specific remedies, and a timely re-evaluation to determine progress.

The physical analysis is taken directly from the pages of functional training, and based on a series of movement screens – such as the aforementioned *overhead squat.* Movement deficiencies (did you: retain balance, tilt to either side, allow your arms to move in front of your body, raise your heels?) are then applied to a grid that matches faults to cures, and identifies strength or stretching exercises to address the client's needs. Unlike traditional fitness evaluations (of strength, flexibility, cardiovascular ability or body fat), a functional analysis is subjective - analogous to a physical therapist identifying problems by watching body parts move.

Once needs have been established, and remedies identified, the program shifts to execution, to the workout itself, which is where its real problems begin.

The Strength Compromise

The hallmark of functional exercise - the combination of strength and skill training - dilutes the strength component due to three factors: choice of equipment, choice of exercises and choice of philosophy.

Choice of Equipment

The props on the studio set of The Golf Channel's *Fitness Academy*, television's version of TPI, dispel any claims of sharpening the tools of golf by strengthening and stretching muscles. Muscles can be stretched without much fanfare, but effective strengthening requires equipment suited for the task. At first glance, the set reminded me of a rehab center in Delray Beach, Florida, that had nothing more than a broomstick to treat chronic back pain. I was accustomed to using a $60,000 machine that accurately measured and strengthened the muscles of the lumbar spine, and wondered, *"How do you strengthen a muscle from thin air?"*

The studio set is equipped with a pulley station, latex bands and free-weights, which allow replication of skill patterns through a variety of movement planes – skills that do *not* transfer to golf. By design, single-station exercise machines are nowhere to be found, a fact not lost on others.

Tim Wakeham, Assistant Strength and Conditioning Coach of the Michigan State Spartans, contests the diminished use and exclusion of exercise machines:

> *Since movements with resistance added to them are no longer replications, does it matter what resistance mode is used for enhancing sport performances? Everything is non-functional when it comes to producing a meaningful (skill) transfer.*
>
> *According to my reading, transfer appears to drop dramatically when even one factor between the training mode and performance differs. Everything from free weights, machines, medicine balls and resistance bands, share many differences when compared to actual sport performance. Some coaches have professed that free weights have a greater ability to produce statistically significant transfer to performance when compared to machines.*
>
> *I'd be interested in reading the definitive, unbiased, valid and reliable research. If a free-weight exercise does transfer more than its machine counterpart, how much more transfer are we talking about? If the free-weight exercise transfers 10% of usable adaptation while the machine transfers 6%, is this a meaningful difference?"*[1]

No such research exists.

I am intrigued by a television ad on The Golf Channel that promotes performance training. From clips that demonstrate the dynamic nature of the exercise movements to the *hands-on* professional attention of the biomechanical experts running the show, the ad grabs the attention of the audience just before it falls flat on its face - when it unveils the *pro-style* fitness tools that form an integral part of the program: Latex bands and Swiss balls. They make training different, special and exciting by allowing movement in paths defined by the user, which satisfies the current trend to have exercise *look* and *feel* like golf.

Years ago, PGA Tour professional, Tom Kite appeared at the MedX® booth of a trade show and was placed on the latest version of the company's torso rotation machine by general manager, Jim Flanagan. Within a few repetitions, he commented, *"Man, this is just like the golf swing."* The TPI program would not allow him near that piece: The use of single-station exercise machines is prohibited.

In a similar manner, Arnold Palmer arrived at the doorstep of Dr. Michael Fulton – then, orthopedic representative for Nautilus Sports/Medical Industries - for an appointment related to a low-back issue. Fulton reviewed Palmer's medical history and imagery, and tested the function of his low-back. The assessment led to an exercise room where the golf legend was placed on several machines with a thorough explanation of how each would address his specific need. The comment he made on the torso rotation machine came as no surprise: *"I think this might add about twenty yards to my drive."*

Both Kite and Palmer recognized that the equipment they were on had the potential to advance their games. They were correct. It didn't hurt that the rotational machines felt *like golf*, despite the fact that their purpose was to isolate and strengthen rotational muscles.

To the point: You must be ill, ill-informed, or naïve, to believe that latex bands and Swiss balls will activate your competitive best in golf. You can find better tools in a broom closet in Delray Beach.

Thirty years ago, the gadgets currently used in golf performance programs would have been laughed out of the building. And that's not all. Every new tool that appears on the exercise scene is quickly adapted to - and adopted by - every sport imaginable. Thus, we have vibration training for golf, yoga for golf, Pilates for golf, gyrotonics for golf, TRX for golf – everything but proper strength training for golf.

The obsession is clear: The direction, skewed.

Choice of Exercises

A second factor that dilutes strength acquisition in functional training is choice of exercises. While multi-joint movements activate more muscle mass, burn more calories during and after exercise, and better stimulate the cardiovascular system than single-joint exercises, their exclusive use makes it difficult to identify weak links in the chain, and determine the contribution of each muscle to the whole. More importantly, it does not allow *any* muscle in the chain to reach its strength potential.

Choice of Philosophy

The third factor relates to training philosophy. High intensity is a prerequisite for best results from strength training – anything less means fewer results. Yet, functional training dictates the performance of exercise *without* intensity to avoid nervous system disruption. If a stronger athlete is a better athlete, as the Nautilus inventor suggests, a functionally-trained athlete is logically something less.

I once asked Jack Nicklaus about the major source of power in the golf swing. *"From the ground up,"* he replied – meaning lower body, leg and hip muscles. The TPI program is more specific. *"Glutes are king,"* they claim - strength in the large muscles of the butt is the key to power and stability in the swing. Few would argue the point, but everyone should challenge the application - the use of *functional* exercises that *prevent* glutes from ever reaching their strength potential. Better choices are available, but involve the use of equipment that remains outside the realm of functional guidelines - no single-joint or single-station exercise machines, and no sitting during the performance of an exercise. The nonsense reminds me of the reluctance of free-weight trainees to use Nautilus machines as they were intended; and in some cases, a reluctance to use them at all.

Fortunately, the dismal functional approach to strengthening glutes may be a blessing, in light of Arthur Jones' take on the prominence of low-back problems in the general population:

> *Weakness in the large muscles of the buttocks and legs is not the problem. On the contrary, the strength of these muscles may be the source of the problem in lower-back injuries. When these larger and far stronger muscles produce a high and dangerous level of force that is imposed on the much weaker muscles of the lumbar area, then you frequently will have a problem.*[2]

The nominal intensity of functional exercise - as performed in the TPI program - is not likely to create back problems, and less likely to prevent them. To add, the program's obsession with small muscle groups that *stabilize* means less training time for muscles that create a greater impact on performance.

The Skill Compromise

One of the underlying principles of functional training is the application of resistance to an established skill - a lousy idea.

When many muscles are involved in the performance of a skill - as they are in the golf swing - the force contribution of each must remain proportionate to the others to retain control of the movement within the confines of the skill. As greater resistance is applied to an established skill, the force within each muscle must increase to preserve the desired proportion, and ultimately, the quality of movement. If the change in resistance is so great that it alters the mechanics of the skill, the proportion of force within each muscle must adapt to accommodate movement efficacy in what has now become a *new* motor program, a different skill.

In other words, you can't practice an ice-hockey skill to improve a golf skill, or vice versa. Yet, this is exactly what occurs in the TPI program.

The Australian research duo of Rushall and Pyke address the importance of specificity as follows:

> *The principle of specificity states that the maximum benefits of a training stimulus can only be obtained when it replicates the movements and energy systems involved in the activities of a sport. This principle may suggest that there is no better training than actually performing in the sport.*[3]

The notion of specificity does not sit well with everyone. *"That abilities are very specific, and that skills do not correlate with each other unless they are virtually identical,"* claims Richard A. Schmidt, Ph.D., *"are often troublesome to students because they do not, at first glance, appear to agree with a number of common observations."*

One observation is that exercise appears to enhance athleticism. But let's be clear: *Only* the general nature of exercise (an increase in muscle mass and strength), *not* its skill-based components (since all actions require unique motor patterns), contributes to greater function in sports.

One of the few exercise machines used in golf performance programs is the multi-use pulley station. Why? It allows you to stand during exercise (a pre-requisite of functional training) and lift resistance in any direction (another pre-requisite), including that of a golf swing. And while most trainers agree that stronger muscles improve performance, many believe that strengthening muscles *as they move through the motion of the sport* is better. Not so. If a trainee performs an exercise *similar* to - but not *exact* to - the activity he or she wants to improve, there is *no* transfer of skill. Changing the conditions under which a task is performed requires significant alteration to underlying abilities, which enables the user to get better at an unrelated task. And, *changing the conditions* appears in many forms: an increase or decrease in resistance, intensity or speed of movement; a change of posture or body-weight distribution due to the applied resistance, intensity or speed modification; performing a target skill while supported by a balance tool ... and on and on.

Nautilus inventor, Arthur Jones hit the nail on the head, *"There are no degrees to specificity ... either you have it or you don't. A movement is utterly specific, or it isn't specific at all."*

He explains:

> *Adding a few ounces to the weight of a basketball will do absolutely nothing in the way of increasing your strength for playing basketball ... but it will certainly mess up your skill at basketball. Adding a few pounds to the weight of a basketball will do very little in the way of increasing your strength ... and it will still have some bad effect on your skill, although not as much as the previous example.*

> *So it is obvious that the closer we come to having specificity (in exercise), the worse off we are ... until and unless we have total specificity, in which case we are simply throwing a normal basketball in our usual fashion; which will increase our skill while doing nothing for our strength.[4]*

I recently introduced the concept of specificity to a retired *golf enthusiast* during successive workouts. The next day - his off-day - I spotted him tugging a twenty-pound weight at a pulley station in an effort to replicate the golf swing through impact. It reminded me of Jimmy Olsen's common inquiry at the end of Superman episodes, *"Clark, how come you're never around when Superman's around?"* Despite the clarity, many find it difficult to distinguish specific from non-specific, struggle to accept the nonexistence of transfer, believe otherwise, or simply don't get it – trainers not excluded.

It makes *no sense* to mix skill and strength training when the skill component makes *zero* contribution to improved performance (because it is a different skill) and dilutes the only productive factor - strength gained through exercise. The sense it makes for those touring the country and spreading such hogwash is monetary.

Training the Un-Trainable

Functional training and the TPI program dedicate a lot of time and energy to genetic abilities that cannot be improved. Abilities such as balance, agility and hand-eye coordination play an important supportive role in golf, which makes it easy to connect every drill or exercise that includes these abilities to the Royal and Ancient game. For example:

- A lateral run through an agility course on the floor *"will improve weight shift during the swing."*
- Slamming a weighted ball to the ground from overhead *"increases the muscle's ability to create speed."*
- The use of a balance tool to challenge an exercise leads to, *"See, your balance has improved,"* implying that balance acquired on the new skill improves balance during the golf swing.

It does not.

One day, a trainer from Mars (she was not from this planet) appeared unannounced in our Jupiter facility. *Balance* was her forte as she demonstrated a slow-motion golf swing while standing on a round foam-roll (a balance device common to gyms). Her performance had a mesmerizing effect on her audience, most of whom spent the next few weeks trying to perfect a skill of no value to golf - unless you carry a foam-roll in your bag, use it during play, and swing slowly.

To further illustrate the myth of transfer, I worked with a retired Hall-of-Fame baseball player who entered our program with the intent of qualifying for *The Senior Tour*. He held a low handicap at a local club and was in excellent condition the day I ran him through a dynamic balance test, as follows:

1. Stand on one leg, perpendicular-to and about two feet from a wall.
2. Without moving that foot, turn your torso to face the wall and touch one of three dots placed at different heights on the wall using the hand furthest from the target.
3. Return your torso and head to the original starting position after each touch.

4. Practice a few times, and then see how many touches you can make in thirty seconds.
5. Switch legs and repeat.

I kept time, counted touches and registered the number of balance losses – a skill in itself.

The average performance for amateur golfers in our program was 12-15 wall touches, with 3-4 balance errors, in thirty seconds. Professionals averaged 25-30 touches, with rare balance loss.

The Hall of Famer could not keep pace. The moment he stood on one leg to begin, he was done. He took his inability to perform the simple task with humor, but was openly embarrassed.

He did not have bad balance. In fact, he demonstrated anything but as one of the best third basemen in MLB history, and displayed great balance during the golf swing (reported by those with whom he played). He simply exhibited poor balance for the challenge that day – a clear demonstration that balance is specific to the task, and does *not* transfer from one skill to another.

Why, you ask, did I bother to evaluate something that can't be improved in the first place? I didn't know better at the time - ignorance. I've since taken a two-shot penalty, read up on the subject and moved on - something the creators of the TPI program have yet to do.

Reaction time, balance, hand-eye coordination and agility are genetically determined.[5]

The stunt combinations that form an integral part of TPI training are both creative and progressive. When a skill is mastered, its successor is further complicated, leading clients to reference the *difficulty* of a workout. Since the program is movement-oriented and shuns intensity, any reference to *difficulty* can be solely attributed to the increased demand of the skills. Hanging over a cliff is tough, but having to exercise as you hang over a cliff - with one eye closed and one toe pointed - is tougher. In *all* cases - apart from any strength gained - the stunts are useless despite their anointed connection to golf.

That's the good news: Some are dangerous to boot. One PGA Tour professional reportedly injured himself when he fell in an attempt to stand on a Swiss ball, something his trainer insisted would improve his balance for golf. The only thing it improved was his view of the 'Exit' sign, which is where he should have bolted in the first place.

The challenge of obscure skills in golf performance programs is not the only danger. Golf is considered a *power* sport, which has led the fitness industry on a never-ending quest to develop power. The common approach is to move quickly during the execution of an exercise – an example of bending physiology to suit the needs of a program, when what is needed is the bending of suits. *Any attempt to demonstrate power during exercise represents the quickest route to the hospital.*

Speed of Movement

Following a highly-touted career at high-school and college - as well as with the US Olympic weightlifting team - Alvin Roy was hired by the San Diego Chargers as a strength coach in 1963, an NFL first. The success of the franchise was instant, and led to Roy's future employment with five professional teams. He soon earned a reputation - of introducing steroids to the league - and narrowly avoided jail.

Because of his perceived success, Roy opened twenty-nine fitness studios around the country, facilities that featured his training techniques, as long as the doors were open. He earned a second reputation of opening gyms, selling long-term memberships and skipping town when the timing was right. During a three year span in his home state of Louisiana, he twice scammed the public using the same building. According to Arthur Jones, that was the good news. *"Later, he was almost solely responsible for one of the worst outrages ever associated with the field of exercise."* Roy convinced coaches and players of the supposed benefits of 'explosive' training.

In the early 1970's, Roy visited Nautilus headquarters in Lake Helen, Florida, flaunting his training ideas. *"I initially assumed that he was simply stupid,"* said Jones, *"that he really believed what he was telling people."* Arthur was wrong. On a visit to the spring-training camp of the Kansas City Chiefs that year, Jones found Roy doing *everything but* 'explosive' training in an effort not to hurt anyone, and *nothing* that would help anyone either. As Jones got to know him, Roy finally admitted that he was *"well aware of the dangers from explosive exercises but still promoted them as gospel because 'that was what coaches wanted to hear.'"*

The rest is history. Today's NFL remains neck deep in the dangerous game of 'explosive' training and the practice has slowly edged its way into golf performance programs.

Let's examine the facts.

The Nautilus inventor routinely demonstrated and measured the forces involved during exercise by connecting a force plate (an oversized bathroom scale) to a large oscilloscope to witness the effect of speed on force output during exercise. In one presentation, MedX general manager, Jim Flanagan mounted the force plate with a 60-pound barbell in hand. At 6'5" and 260 pounds, Jim started moving the weight slowly from shoulder height to overhead, and back.

Figure 1: Slow Speed of Movement   Figure 2: Fast Speed of Movement

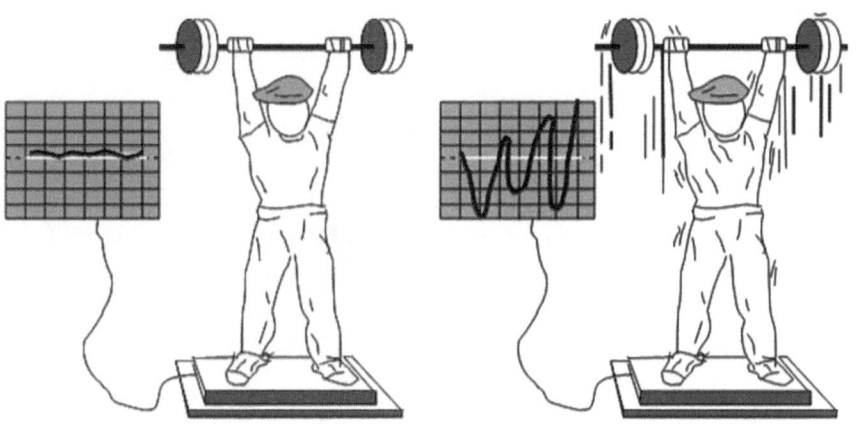

The resistance on the screen - at a slow speed (Figure 1) - remained close to its original value, fifty-eight to sixty-two pounds. Jim steadily increased the speed of movement and eventually slammed the weight up and down above his head. The once-smooth wave left the screen, top and bottom (Figure 2). The thrust of the barbell from Jim's shoulder-height registered a force that exceeded 200 pounds, more than three times its original weight - a dangerous level when joint tolerance is unknown. In other words, *lifting weights rapidly is not safe ... and not productive*. The initial jerk creates momentum that allows muscles to ride through the remainder of the range of motion without performing much, if any, work. In this case, the 60-pound barbell weighed less than zero for more than half the movement. It was literally lifting his arms.

I highlight this for a reason: Functional training and golf performance programs are rooted in the belief that the element of power is best trained by rapid-speed exercise. They are not alone.

Donald Chu, spokesperson for the National Strength and Conditioning Association (NSCA) sums up the consensus. *"Specificity of training tells us that if you train slowly, you move slowly, and if you desire to increase speed of movement you had better include speed training in your program."*[6]

Jones called it his way: *"Hogwash, pure unadulterated garbage, utterly false and dangerously misleading misinformation."* Explosive movement speed during exercise was one of the *fables* he exposed in his 1977 article on specificity: *"How fast one moves while performing exercises for the purpose of building strength,"* he said, *"has absolutely nothing to do with how fast one can move while using the strength of those same muscles."*[7]

To add, a rapid speed of movement during exercise makes no logical sense. If you add weight to an exercise, speed of movement is automatically decreased: Nothing else is possible. You can lift ten pounds quickly, 100 pounds less quickly and your car, not quickly at all. So, how can Chu and others claim to *increase* speed of movement in a task by practicing at a speed that is slower than normal (due to the added resistance)? Did he not claim that slow training results in slow movement?

Slow movement during exercise increases the potential to gain strength through a full range of motion (depending on choice of equipment); and strength increases the potential to generate force. Therefore, the *slower* you move in the gym during exercise, the *faster* you will move on the field.

Not everyone agrees. Baseball pitchers, for example, routinely perform explosive chest (or shoulder) presses with light-to-moderate weights to increase throwing velocity. If the resistance used for such exercise weighs more than a baseball (and it generally does), the practice only serves to *decrease* the speed of movement during exercise compared to that of throwing a baseball. And what does it do for the skill of throwing? Anywhere from *nothing* to *you wouldn't want to know.*

The same can be said of swinging a weighted golf club before play. A few swings may serve as a gentle warm-up, but repetitive swings used as a means to strengthen muscles is not the way to go. Short-term, you'll lose a few golf balls; long term, you may lose hard-earned skill.

Ultimate Speed®, a company that once rented space within our facility in Jupiter, Florida was owned and frequented by a prominent golf-teaching professional who would have better served his clientele by staying home. His highly-educated staff was no better. One day, a director with a Master of Science degree sat a teen on a MedX® chest-press machine with clear instructions, "*Explode*," and seconds later, "***Explode***." While that echoed in my left ear, advice from Arthur Jones resonated in my right. "*The next time somebody suggests that you move suddenly during any form of exercise or testing, smile and walk away, because you are talking to a fool. And do not overlook the fact that a very long list of fools has large muscles, and another long list of fools has all sorts of academic credentials.*"

Like Jim Flanagan, the teen exposed his muscles to high forces upon initiating the exercise, and did little work beyond.

Despite the obvious, many trainers and athletes claim to extract the desired training effect (increased speed on the field) from 'explosive' training, but that may be skewed:

> *Grabe and Widule (1988) determined that much of the training effect from explosive power training is due to the motor learning of the skill associated with the activity. The actual activities of the sport would seem to be the best training exercises for the development of both speed and power.*[8] And (from the same source) ...

> *Training for power and speed would seem to be relatively simple. The activity itself should form the basis of the form of movement, the technique should be as economical as possible, and given the*

restrictions of this, the action should be as intense as possible. Anything less than a maximum effort will train different neuromuscular patterns and should be considered counterproductive.[9]

The formula to increase speed of movement and *power* on the golf course is simple:

- Increase your skill.
- Increase the strength of the muscles involved.
- Keep strength training *independent* of skill training.
- Decrease overall body fat (to reduce friction during muscle contraction).

The Ultimate Insult: Plyometrics

One afternoon, NBA Hall-of-Fame player and coach, Bill Cunningham and I watched the 'experts' from Ultimate Speed® attach a high-school athlete to a device designed to increase vertical jump. The *Power Jumper* connected a platform base to the waist of the trainee by a series of latex tubes to facilitate vertical leaps against resistance. *"During my playing days,"* Cunningham chuckled, *"we had a salesman drop by to promote a similar device. Coach agreed to give it a try, so we used it several times a week after practice."* To the point: The team's ability to jump was significantly reduced, while Bill lost *"several inches."*

Rushall and Pyke explain:

> *Adjustments to technique to handle the minor loads (of extra-load training) might produce negative training effects because of the subtle alteration to refined neuromuscular movement patterns. Extra-load resistances used on the extremities have not been shown to be of value for training.[10]*

Sports-performance advocates insist that 'explosive' movements and plyometric activities (jumping on or over boxes from various levels, jump squats, etc.) are safe and productive; and that their programs follow the SAID principle (Specific Adaptation to Imposed Demand) to the letter.

Their logic is simple - *to prepare the body for the high forces of impact* (in sports), *you must expose it to, or practice, impact* (such as that encountered during plyometric activities). That's the equivalent of telling an athlete to continue to smoke to prepare his or her body for the high price it will eventually pay.

During a conference in the early 1970's, a biomechanical expert spoke of the high and dangerous levels of impact-force associated with jogging. Twenty minutes later, he recommended jump squats as a safe and productive alternative. It was his second error: Arthur Jones was in the audience. *"The level of impact force involved in jogging,"* blurted Jones, *"is usually about three times as high as the subject's bodyweight, but with jump squats it may be fifty times as high as bodyweight. So, if jogging is dangerous, how in the hell can jump squats be safe?"*

Jones knew. He routinely measured the phenomenon at the MedX complex in Ocala, Florida using his force plate and oscilloscope.

He generally began by seeking a volunteer - prompting the ill-informed to rush to their demise. On one occasion, a six-foot, 200-pound running-back mounted the plate, which produced a force of 200 pounds on the screen. Jones asked the young man to jog lightly on the spot, whereupon his effort registered a force of 600 pounds at each landing. Arthur then instructed the youth to jump approximately four inches high with both feet and land normally. The force plate registered one thousand pounds, five times his bodyweight. Not good.

Tiger Woods

In a recent interview, Tiger Woods commented that he felt more 'explosive' every day in his recovery from back surgery.

He was, by design.

Muscle atrophy - the aftermath of surgery - affects a muscle's powerful, fast-twitch fibers more than its endurance–oriented, slow-twitch fibers. As a muscle strengthens and recovers, the fast-twitch fibers gradually resume their normal proportion and role - that of facilitating explosive movement in sports – as a natural part of the healing process. That alone makes Tiger Woods more 'explosive' every day of his recovery.

Training muscle to become explosive by maximizing speed of movement *during* exercise would expedite a return to the hospital.

In a similar action, Tiger Woods was forced to jump down into a bunker following a difficult stance and swing at the 2014 Bridgestone Invitational in Akron, Ohio. His return to competitive golf from recent low-back surgery was thwarted by the force of impact during the jump – a force that proved greater than the strength of his back, and much greater than what he had encountered during the swing.

Few trainers and coaches have been privy to the analogies Arthur Jones used to convey the danger of impact during plyometric training:

- *"Jump from your bathroom vanity onto your scale to see how much you weigh. In the air you'll weigh nothing; when you land, you might weigh several thousand pounds."*
- *"Plyometrics is the equivalent of running your athletes to the top of the stadium stairs and having them jump into the parking lot."*
- *"Anyone dumb enough to do plyometrics will get exactly what they deserve – hurt."*

Not everyone agrees. *"To deny the effects of plyometric (explosive) training,"* claims Donald Chu, *"is to deny the obvious."* What obvious?

The obvious was clearly demonstrated - in my face - by Jim Flanagan: *One*, that 'fast' exposes the involved muscles to high and dangerous levels of force; *Two*, that strength gains are minimized by an explosive speed of movement due to momentum; and *Three*, that the *only* direct result of explosive training is injury.

Why, then, is *explosive* exercise included in golf programs?

Besides an attempt to satisfy the *power* component of golf through contemporary means, TPI program proponents believe that rapid movement against resistance activates a muscle's powerful fast-twitch fibers. It does not. Fast-twitch fibers are activated by intensity of effort, which means they are not likely to be activated at all in lieu of functional training's evasive stance on intensity.

To add insult to pending injury, the impact encountered during plyometric activities in the gym is *different* than that encountered on the field. And different means *non-specific*. Exposure to plyometric activity A, for example, results in the body's adaptation to the demands of plyometric activity A. Exposure to plyometric activity B results in adaptation to the demands of plyometric activity B, and so on. Other than the strength gained through the practice of plyometric activities (which is compromised by momentum), plyometrics does *not* prepare the body for the demands of impact encountered on the field. Each impact on a football field, for example, is unique - different forces at different angles imposed on different body parts - which makes specific preparation impossible. The only thing that prepares the body for the demands of impact is strength – increasing the integrity of muscle and joint systems to resist force. The assumption of transfer from plyometric activities to sports performance does *not* exist – which makes many training traditions look foolish.

In the field of exercise, blame lies with national certification organizations that create their own version of physiology and aggressively recruit interested candidates - including TPI trainers. The result:

> *Most of the millions of people who are now interested in exercise are too young to even be aware of the true history of this field, do not know who to believe or what to believe, remain unaware of the many outrages that have occurred during the past 50 years or so in this field, many of which outrages are still occurring. Outrages? You're damned right: isokinetics, plyometrics, power cleans, any sudden movement against resistance, jump squats and a long list of other things that provide no benefits whatsoever and are dangerous as hell.*[11]

Why should golfers be exposed to impact?

They shouldn't: Impact should remain in the hands of teaching professionals, and limited to the bottom of the swing.

Conclusion

The application of functional training to the high-skill sport of golf – embodied by the TPI program - will not produce a happy ending:

- It hinders skill by violating the concept of *specificity* through replication of sports movements against resistance.

- It hampers strength gains by limiting work intensity, and restricting the choice of tools and exercises to those that provide inferior resistance to the working muscles.
- It encourages 'explosive' speed of movement during exercise, and introduces athletes to the ultimate insanity, impact. Both lead to nothing but injury.

The common response to the above is defensive. Many TPI trainers claim to identify, strengthen and stretch muscles used in the swing without attempting to replicate golf movements against resistance. If you give them the benefit of the doubt – and I won't – why is the program as physically recognizable and as inept as it appears?

The nervous system does *not* question a muscle's source of strength during its moment of need. It doesn't care whether you used free weights, machines or rubber bands to gain strength; whether you stood, sat, kneeled or snored during the strength-acquisition stage; whether strength was gained in a single or multiple-movement plane; or whether you trained by replicating the golf swing or not. The nervous system only asks a muscle to contribute to the effort by means of a force input at a precise moment – and hopes the request can be honored. It is less likely to be honored if the mindset and application of functional training continues its meteoric rise.

The press hasn't helped.

In a 2014 discussion on the status of Tiger Woods' low back after surgery, The Golf Channel's Tim Rosafort commented: *"Tiger needs to drop the heavy lifting and turn more in the direction of golf-specific training."* Whether he knows anything about the topic or not, Rosafort is entitled to an opinion. Unfortunately, when that opinion reaches a broad television audience, it bears significant weight. I can only hope that the date of the broadcast was equally significant, April 1.

Like fellow-Canadian, Moe Norman, I like quality, and I like simple. Moe became so proficient at hitting a golf ball straight that he thought it was easy, and couldn't understand why others didn't find it so. When asked about his approach to the game, he said in all sincerity, *"Here's the ball. There's the hole. Play."* And when asked about his ball-striking prowess, he replied, *"Easy. Just hit this stupid thing* (pointing to a ball on the ground), *with this stupid thing* (pointing to a club) *into that stupid thing* (pointing to a hole)." His response helped no one, but provided insight into his perception of the game. Lack of anxiety and freedom from thought allowed his body to do what it was capable of, every time.

A quality physical approach to golf can, and should, be simple: 8-10 basic exercises, twice a week, 15-20 minutes per session.

More than a decade ago, I wrote a brief article about the signature eighth hole at my home course. It conveys a timely message:

Presbyterian Pass

As a teen, I gave no thought to the fact that my first set of golf clubs consisted of wooden-shafted hand-me-downs, my brother's paper-route Christmas bonus from a prominent Judge in town. Despite the hockey-tape that held them together, one club - a putter made in the mid-1920's - performed nobly enough to keep. To this day, it retains its stature in an upgraded set, ignoring sneers of 'old-fashioned' from its victims.

At the same time, I gave little thought to the proposed modification of the golf course we played. The Board of Directors claimed a few holes were unfair - the greens were not receptive to good shots and often rewarded bad ones. They were right to some extent, but dead wrong in the case of the eighth.

It wasn't length or degree of difficulty that made the eighth a world-class hole. At 150 yards from the lower tee and 185 from the tip of the upper, it could play anywhere from a feathered nine-iron to a screaming driver, depending on the wind. It was 'character.'

The Lookout Point Golf Club in Fonthill, Ontario was built in 1922 on the edge of the Niagara Escarpment, a rock formation that left dramatic rifts in elevation throughout the area. The clubhouse sat atop "the highest point on the Peninsula" and overlooked the spray from Niagara Falls in one direction, the Toronto skyline in the other and seven holes below. Only two challenged the escarpment. The par-four eighteenth abandoned its attempt half way up, from where a much needed cable-car ride intervened. The par-three eighth, aptly named Presbyterian Pass, provided no such ease.

The narrow path that climbed to the eighth began at the base of a dense-wooded hill. At the tee, the bush succumbed to an array of grassy sumac-strewn hills that intertwined as fingers in a clasp of hands. The tee itself cut into the left side of the first hill that ushered in a series of progressively ascending slopes cascading from left, then right, then left - neither side friendly to an errant shot. At their feet, a swath of fairway wound its way to an elevated green nestled between two final mounds whose grassy tops hovered 30 feet above the putting surface. The green was flanked by a shallow bunker etched into the face of each hill, a craggy sumac protruding above the one on the right.

The climb was steep, the shot dangerous. Anything short rolled back 20-30 yards. Long flirted with a deep but elevated grass bunker from which there was no reasonable escape. In the summer months, when the grass was dry, a wayward shot bounded from the hillsides toward the green. It was the only way to get close.

In the end, they leveled the hill left of the green, enlarged the putting surface to uncharacteristic proportions, gently sloped its entrance and filled in the grass bunker.

Presbyterian Pass, once in a class with the Postage Stamp at Royal Troon, the 9th at Jupiter Hills and the Alps at Prestwick, was built by U.S. and British Amateur champion, Walter Travis, author of his own (Schenectady) putter controversy in 1904. Remodel it? As Bernard Darwin wrote in The Golf Courses of the British Isles, *1910, about proposed changes to Royal St. George's Golf Club (England), "Why do they want to alter this adorable place? I know they are perfectly right, and I have even agreed with them that this is a blind shot and that an indefensively bad hole, but what does it all matter? This is perfect bliss."*

To walk its path in the fall, to set spikes on its tee in a breeze, to behold its rugged beauty and challenge its rigors was indeed 'perfect bliss.' One day, someone will see fit to restore the eighth to its original state and I'll be first to donate a shovel.[12]

I like quality, and I like simple: The TPI program is neither. Like the famous eighth at Lookout Point, traditional training for golf does *not* require an overhaul. But its successor – golf performance training – could surely benefit from my proposed donation.

References

1. Brian Johnston, *System Analysis* (Sudbury, ON: Bodyworx Publishing, 2001), 173.
2. Arthur Jones, "The Requirements for Meaningful Testing of Lumbar Function," *Risk & Benefits Management,* November (1987).
3. B.S. Rushall and F.S. Pyke, *Training for Sports and Fitness* (Melbourne, Australia: Macmillan of Australia, 1991).
4. Arthur Jones, "Specificity in Strength Training ... The Facts and Fables," *Athletic Journal,* May (1977).
5. Brian Johnston, *System Analysis* (Sudbury, ON: Bodyworx Publishing, 2001), 137.
6. Brian Johnston, *System Analysis* (Sudbury, ON: Bodyworx Publishing, 2001), 158.
7. Arthur Jones, "Preventing Injuries in Sports," *Athletic Journal,* May (1975).
8. B.S. Rushall and F.S. Pyke, *Training for Sports and Fitness* (Melbourne, Australia: Macmillan of Australia, 1991).
9. B.S. Rushall and F.S. Pyke, *Training for Sports and Fitness* (Melbourne, Australia: Macmillan of Australia, 1991).
10. B.S. Rushall and F.S. Pyke, *Training for Sports and Fitness* (Melbourne, Australia: Macmillan of Australia, 1991).
11. Arthur Jones, "My First Half Century in the Iron Game," Ironman, November (1993), 190.
12. Gary Bannister, *In Arthur's Shadow* (Carmel, IN: Cork Hill Press, 2005), 452.

Hole #9: 522 Yards, Par 5

FUNCTIONAL TRAINING VS TRADITIONAL TRAINING

My initial contact with functional training occurred when the fitness/rehabilitation facility in which I worked hired physical therapist, Jessica Parnevik to help establish a golf training program. Jessica, the sister of an established star on the PGA Tour, had great credentials and an outstanding personality for a high-profile clientele. Her introduction to the staff came in the form of a presentation on the benefits of functional training.

The golf program was three-pronged: A PGA professional handled the skill component; Jessica supervised functional exercise; and I was responsible for strength training. We coordinated efforts - yet retained the freedom to do *our thing* - and focused on the quality of the product.

The response was overwhelming, but my brief, visual contact with functional training left lingering doubts about its contribution. My studies at McMaster University and the writings of Arthur Jones had shaped my thought process.

When I finally put the puzzle together, it was like a long drive down the fairway. The combination of skill and strength training in an exercise setting could not work - was of no value from the skill perspective, and not much better from the strength side. Besides that, it challenged the system's ability to process information: Did the brain require assistance to connect the strength of a muscle to the skill of a task? Did strength need a hand-held stroll down a nervous system pathway to learn its proper application? Was the nervous system incapable of solving a puzzle on its own, as it had *before* the arrival of functional training? And more global: "What did functional training add to the mix?" and "How did it stack up to traditional training?"

Hole #2 discussed the potential benefits of exercise from a traditional approach. Let's briefly examine the same benefits from a functional perspective, with apologies - minor repetition is inevitable.

Strength

Functional-training's focus on movement rather than on muscles that produce movement, results in poor strength gains:

1. Functional tools of choice are limited to those that allow body parts to move in any plane or direction. This restriction fails to:
    - apply resistance directly to the working muscles,
    - match the resistance to the changing needs of a muscle as it moves and ...
    - deliver a challenging overload to a muscle in full-contraction.

    ... in brief, it eliminates the possibility of full-range exercise.

2. Functional exercise performed in a non-stable environment limits the amount of resistance one can use. Years ago, I exercised on a set of Cybex® *Dual Axis* machines that were, I was warned, *"dangerous as hell"* - the movement arms were free to roam in user-defined paths, an attempt to compete in the 'unrestricted-movement' domain. Without the skill to control the movement, I was forced to reduce the resistance to feel safe. Yet, what experts hailed a plus (that reduced stability forces *stabilizers* to support working muscles), Arthur Jones hailed a minus. *"The only thing likely to happen,"* he said, *"is injury to the 'balancing' muscles."* Ironically, the warning label on the *Dual-Axis* machines states: *Arms move in paths directed by user. Incorrect path can cause injury. Movement must be controlled in proper path.* Wonderful. The manufacturer trusts the user to select a path they are unwilling to identify - not

a problem. From every path, the logic behind instability training for strength is weak: *Why use a resistance high enough to stimulate muscle growth when you can use less and stimulate nothing?*

3. The exclusive use of exercises that involve multiple joints is burdened by its own problems. Often, the weak link in the work-chain is either overloaded, which results in growth stimulation or injury; or bypassed, which does nothing to address the weakness. In addition, multi-joint exercise inhibits the involved muscles from achieving their strength and range-of-motion potentials. When a muscle cannot reach full-contraction, where all of its fibers are involved, maximum strength gains are impossible. When it cannot reach full extension, flexibility increases are equally impossible.

4. By design, functional exercise avoids intensity, a component vital to strength gain. Arthur Jones once warned with a finger in my face, "*If you do ten repetitions of an exercise when you could have done twelve, you may as well stay in the parking lot … you'll get the same result – nothing.*" Functional training will keep you in the parking lot.

It gets worse. Movement-based training, regardless of intensity, provides a stimulus that is insufficient to *maintain* strength:

> *Carlile and Carlile (1961) reported that Australian swimmers trained with weight exercises prior to commencing hard swimming training in preparation for an Olympic Games. During the swimming training, no weight training was performed. After 10 weeks of swimming training that produced over-trained states, thereby attesting to the intensity of the training load, it was found that strength gains that had previously been achieved prior to swimming had regressed back to untrained levels.*[1]

Flexibility

The exclusive use of multi-joint exercises in functional training does not allow muscles to reach positions where stretching can occur, which results in flexibility loss.

Cardiovascular Condition

Cardiovascular benefits gained through traditional versus functional means are similar, but inconclusive. When exercise is performed with no rest between efforts, the intensity and quality of resistance favors traditional training. On the other hand, the quantity of muscle mass involved in multi-joint exercise favors functional training. A study conducted in 1975 may tip the scale.

The greatest cardiovascular result in the history of exercise was produced during *Project Total Conditioning,* an experiment at the US Military Academy in West Point, NY. The strength-training program, orchestrated by Arthur Jones, produced cardiovascular results that Dr. Kenneth Cooper's aerobic staff could not believe – and they measured them. Ironically, the results were produced by a football team as they *sat on exercise machines* – a functional no-no. Details on Hole #13.

Compared to the other potential benefits of exercise, cardiovascular improvement may be the best, if not the only result of a well-designed functional program. Once again, how critical is it to golf?

Body Composition

Functional exercise makes a poor contribution to the reduction of body fat because it fails to stimulate significant muscle mass. The most efficient way to reduce body fat is to increase the amount of muscle on your body - a concept foreign to a system that focuses on movement. As a result, the effect of functional training, properly performed, is greater on the cardiovascular than the muscular system, leaving trainees with body-composition results similar to those produced by cardiovascular activity – a loss of bodyweight from muscle, organ and fat tissue.

Injury Prevention

Injury prevention, for the most part, depends on the strength of muscles, connective tissue and bones that comprise the joint.

Functional advocates stress the importance of strong joint stabilizers and believe that injury is more related to *faulty movement patterns* than weak structural support. They criticize the fixed path and balanced resistance provided by exercise machines, without acknowledging that heavy free-weight and functional exercises have their own fixed path. At the same time, they ignore the strength of the large muscles that surround the joint, as well as injuries caused by the application of force to a muscle/joint system as it operates in an unstable environment.

The stability increase claimed by the acquisition of skill in performing functional exercise is inferior to the stability acquired through stronger muscles. Increased strength protects you from injury; enhanced skill through unrelated movement-training does not.

Summary

Regardless of claims, functional exercise *cannot* help trainees reach their functional potential:

- It minimizes the role of strength - the only productive factor in performance.
- It promotes flexibility loss by adhering to multi-joint exercises.
- It can trigger a significant cardiovascular response, but is rarely performed with high intensity and minimal rest between efforts.
- It provides a poor stimulus to modify body-composition.
- Strength, more than proper movement, prevents injury.

Research

Let's examine conclusions from studies that applied *functional* concepts to athletic performance.

1. Swimmers who trained against additional resistance in the pool:

   "Costill, Sharp, and Troup (1980) concluded that swimming strength is best achieved by repeated maximum exercises that duplicate as

closely as possible the skill of swimming. The most appropriate exercise that they suggested was a series of maximum sprint swims."[2]

Repetition of the exact skill is superior to repetition of something 'like' the skill.

2. Summer training for speed skaters:

    ... *"neither low walking (walking-like movement in skating position) nor dry skating (side-to-side, deep sitting push-offs) can be considered as specific training activities for speed skaters. There are no valuable training effects that will enhance speed skating from the enactment of these activities. They are useless activities for competent skaters. They could even be counter-productive if emphasized too heavily (probably would cause disruption of high-level neuromuscular patterns).*"[3]

If these activities were useless thirty years ago, why are they in popular use today?

3. The effect of modified resistance on swimming mechanics (paraphrased):

    Four male and two female groups were filmed as they sprinted the butterfly (approximately 40 feet) under three conditions: one, normally; two, partially resisted (tethered by a swim belt); and three, sprint-assisted using a tethered belt. A biomechanical analysis revealed the following: ONE, sprint-resisted training caused a shorter and slower stroke; TWO, sprint-assisted training increased the stroke rate (by shortening stroke length, not changing hand velocity); THREE, stroke mechanics were changed in both forms of training, casting doubt on their efficacy; and FOUR, this study should be considered an indictment of these training methods. Each method encouraged swimmers to adopt less efficient mechanics.[4]

The use of an overload or under-load during the performance of a skill changes the mechanics of the skill. Yet, it is precisely what occurs when golf performance programs attempt to replicate movement patterns against resistance. Skill is a key component of functional ability and performance, but - unless weightlifting is your sport - it is not a potential benefit of exercise.

4.   An observation:

Ask a football coach about his team's first practice in full or partial uniform. The coordination and timing of plays without pads is suddenly upset by the weight of what the athletes wear - they are slower; the team, slower. The added resistance disrupts the skill established in shirt sleeves.

Adding resistance to a skill or movement pattern does not strengthen or reinforce the movement pattern. It creates a new and different skill.

Conclusion

The benefits of functional exercise applied to sports are limited to two effects: a cardiovascular response and the acquisition of unrelated skills. Claims of improved performance by its participants may be sincere, but extend to *any* form of exercise:

- Overloading a muscle can produce a benefit, and functional training provides an overload – a poor one, but an overload nonetheless.
- The different challenge provided by functional training might motivate trainees to work hard and produce a greater net effect that extends to their skill training.
- Many trainees practice traditional, functional and skill training at the same time, making it impossible to determine specific contributions.

Despite the perception that functional training works for those not willing or able to do something better, the popularity of the approach has inundated the field of exercise with trainers who are unaware of the simplicity of what they are trying to accomplish. An increase in performance, as it relates to muscle function and its corresponding application to sports, requires one of two things (or both):

1. *An increase in skill.* The continual practice of an exercise (or movement) produces greater lifting proficiency (or skill). The establishment of neuromuscular patterns through practice enhances the ability to lift weights (or perform tasks) in a safer, more efficient manner.

2. *An increase in strength (or lean muscle mass).* Muscle gained through proper strength training increases joint stability, and the ability to generate and resist force. Such increase can be stimulated by various means - free weights, bodyweight exercise, machines and Swiss-ball movements - but is *not* exclusive to so-called functional-training exercise.

Jesper Parnevik and his sister, Jessica, produced a functional-exercise golf video well in advance of entering our facility. Years ago, I caught up with him at a restaurant that hosted our year-end staff party. I hadn't seen him in a decade, and was flattered by a comment. *"Hey. Remember the training we did, that one-set-to-failure stuff you had us do? I think I got my best results with that."* I recently viewed his private gym, and can only hope he employs a system on par with his equipment.

Despite the obvious shortcomings of their system, functional-exercise advocates are dedicated to their craft. *"If you had to rate bodybuilding exercises for their average level of motor complexity on a scale of ten, ten being very complex,"* states author, Paul Chek, *"then a score of 1-4 would be fair."* Nice speech, considering that the relationship between the value of a highly complex exercise and functional improvement has *never* been established, and *never will,* due to the unique nature of skills and abilities within each task. If I had to rate the contribution of functional exercise (*versus* traditional exercise) to potential benefits and performance on a similar scale, my scores would also be *fair,* as follows:

Figure 1: Functional Exercise versus Traditional Exercise

Contribution of ➡	Functional Ex.	Traditional Ex.
To: Strength	1-4	10
Flexibility	0	7-10
Cardiovascular Condition	7-10	8-10
Body Composition	1-3	8-10
Injury Prevention	1-4	10
Skill	0	0

… and the experts have the audacity to call movement training, *functional*? It adds nothing to the skill component of performance, and makes a dismal contribution to the only productive benefit of exercise – muscle strength.

I stood on the par-three 8th tee of the Olde Mill Golf Club in Laurel Fork, Virginia, in 1974. A ten-year-old boy I caught up to during play kindly allowed me to play through. The hole demanded a lengthy carry over a rugged ravine to a shallow green. I considered two clubs and made the critical selection. The ball flew high and straight, descending on a line just left of the pin. As I posed to admire my effort, the ball disappeared deep into the jagged ravine beyond the green. When the smoke cleared, the kid spoke up, *"Nice shot, Mister. You just got a bad result."*

And so it is with those who choose functional training (in this case, the TPI program) as their ticket to a lower handicap. You can do everything right along the way and ultimately end with *a bad result.*

Why bother?

The Back Nine begins with a three-hole stretch – my *Amen Corner* – that examines, in depth, concepts and tools (or lack thereof) common to golf performance training. It may open a few eyes.

References

1. B.S. Rushall and F.S. Pyke, *Training for Sports and Fitness* (Melbourne, Australia: Macmillan of Australia, 1991).
2. B.S. Rushall and F.S. Pyke, *Training for Sports and Fitness* (Melbourne, Australia: Macmillan of Australia, 1991).
3. R.W. De Boer et al., "Specific Characteristics of Speed Skating: Implications for Summer Training," *Medicine and Science in Sports and Exercise* 19 (1987), 504.
4. E.W. Maglischo et al., "The Effects of Sprint-Assisted and Sprint-Resisted Swimming on Stroke Mechanics," *Journal of Swimming Research* 1 (1985), 27.

BACK NINE

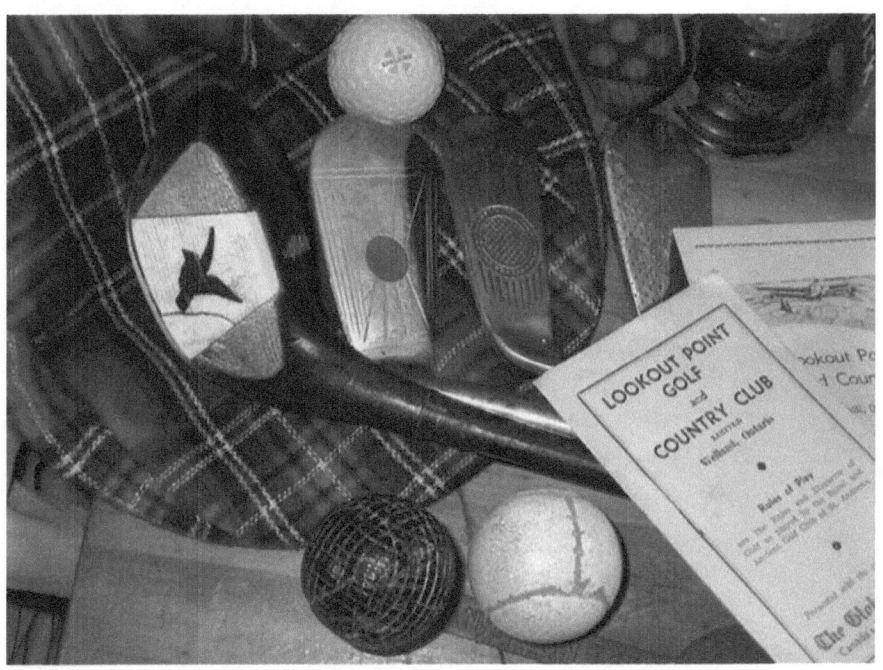

IN

Hole #10: 435 Yards, Par 4

CORE TRAINING

Research conducted a half-century ago determined that the muscles of the lumbar spine were stronger than those of the abdomen - strength determined by the amount of electrical activity in a muscle: The greater the activity, the stronger the muscle. The studies resulted in the development of a series of abdominal exercises - commonly known as William's flexion exercises - to balance the discrepancy between front and rear torso muscles. The protocol was adopted by the medical community, proved successful in the treatment of chronic low-back pain, and spawned the advice I heard every time I visited a specialist, *Strengthen your abdomen.* I did.

Shortly thereafter, a physical therapist from New Zealand named Robin McKenzie claimed to produce significant results in pain perception by exposing his patients to extension exercises (rather than flexion) to strengthen the muscles of the rear torso. His approach was more direct: Back problem? Strengthen back muscles. The medical community eventually determined that certain diagnoses responded better to flexion exercises; others, to extension.

Treatment solutions for chronic back pain had improved, but were far from written in stone.

In 1972, Arthur Jones began to construct a tool to isolate and accurately measure the strength of the muscles that extend the spine (the same reportedly measured a half-century before). His mission was clear: *Total muscle isolation.* Fourteen years later, he introduced a device that was nominated for a Nobel Prize in medicine. In the process, he tested approximately ten thousand subjects and found the majority in a state of what he called *chronic disuse atrophy* - they had never used those muscles.

He concluded that lumbar extensor muscles, not abdominals, were the weak link.

A decade of research at the University of Florida and the University of California at San Diego supported Jones' contention and confirmed the need to strengthen the muscles that extend the spine. Jones stood tall on two points. *One*: The day he announced, *"Gentlemen, abdominal strength has nothing to do with low-back pain,"* I thought the orthopedic surgeons in the room would fall out of their chairs. *Two*: He followed with, *"Traditional exercise for lumbar extensors is useless for its intended purpose."* Arthur loved the value of shock, but was more enamored with truth.

As this unfolded, I witnessed my own sideshow – the arrival of core training: *"The balanced development of the superficial muscles that stabilize, align and move the trunk of the body, especially the abdominals and muscles of the back."*[1] It sprung to the forefront in the same manner as functional training: Someone woke up one morning and declared *the core* important – for everyday activities, for posture, for aesthetics, for sports and, last but not least, for money. Overnight, it became the missing piece of the puzzle. Gym floors crawled with clients performing high-school exercises they once despised, competing for space around equipment they once used.

It took me by surprise, and I knew it would gravitate to golf.

The connection was clear: In simple terms, the core consists of three muscle groups that surround the torso - abdominals in front, lumbar muscles in back, and obliques on the sides. In golf, core muscles connect a relatively stable base (the lower body) to an active upper body, and strength between the two contributes to performance, delays the onset of fatigue and helps prevent injury. Core strength is vital to success, claim the experts, and the frenzy extends from recreational golfers to tour professionals, from greens-keepers to television announcers, from teaching pros to scorekeepers.

The other side of the coin …

Other than a handful of Joe Blows reporting better golf since they strengthened their *core*, there is no proof - not one objective study - to suggest that a core-trained athlete is a better athlete, or that training the core has improved a golfer's ability to swing more efficiently or effectively. There are too many variables ... but none in what follows:

- Most, if not all, muscles of the body are active in a golf swing, which means that strength gained in *any* muscle should have a positive effect on performance; and may, in turn, justify the reported success of those who train core muscles.
- The ability to generate club-head speed (power) in golf depends more on the contribution of large muscle groups than small. Core training has become so important that 20-30 minutes of exclusive core exercise is common, often at the expense of large-muscle work.
- Approximately 80 percent of people suffer low-back pain in their lifetime, which supports the claim that the most important muscles of the core are those that extend the spine (few people suffer abdominal or oblique issues). Yet, most core programs feature a surplus of abdominal exercise compared to that of the low-back - not the *balanced* approach they champion.
- And more important, traditional exercise (including McKenzie's, above) *cannot* meaningfully strengthen the muscles that extend the spine. More on Hole # 11.

The Core and The Tour

A four-year study conducted by Centinela Hospital and a statistical follow-up by their successor, HealthSouth®, revealed that 46 percent of PGA, LPGA and Senior Tour professionals utilized the services of the fitness vans for *low-back problems*, the major issue on tour. Most injuries were first treated using traditional modalities - ice, heat, rest, ultra sound, electrical stimulation and stretching. Once players were symptom-free, the next step – to strengthen spinal muscles – was ignored through no fault of their own. The low-back machines in the vans were not up to par.

Around that time, the University of Florida completed a research study[2] that clearly demonstrated the ineffectiveness of both the Cybex® Eagle back machine (the one in the fitness vans) and the Nautilus® Lower Back machine (commonly used in fitness and rehab centers). Neither had *any* effect on the strength of the muscles that extend the spine. According to the study, both machines allowed the pelvis to rotate, which activated and strengthened muscles of the hip (glutes and hamstrings), with little or no transfer to muscles of the lumbar spine.

The same study compared the results of the Cybex and Nautilus machines to those of a device that *did not* allow the pelvis to rotate, the MedX Lumbar Extension machine (built by Jones). The dramatic improvement in strength of the totally-isolated muscles that extend the spine took the research staff at the University of Florida - as well as thousands of athletes and patients exposed to the brief, infrequent exercise protocol - by surprise. The success of the new device continued for two decades, until those who could best promote the tool turned the other cheek. *"The machine threatened the medical community,"* claimed those involved with its development. *"It might have put them out of business."*

It was a major blow for low-back care, but not the only hurdle a needy group of golf professionals faced.

Twenty years ago, I called HealthSouth® representative, Barry Sommerville, who was in charge of the fitness vans for all three tours and asked what they had for low-backs. *"Each van,"* he said, *"is equipped with an exercise tool to strengthen the spine."* I told him about the results of a study at the University of Florida that was not kind to his selection of a Cybex® Eagle back machine. I mentioned the MedX® tool, but Sommerville claimed he had never heard the name, and was diplomatic. *"HealthSouth remains open to the latest technological advancements,"* he replied. *"Please forward a copy of what you have."* I didn't bother: HealthSouth had a longstanding equipment affair with Cybex® that ensured the vans would be nothing more than first-aid stops for acute pain.

The solution is as clear today as it was then: Install a MedX Lumbar Extension machine in each van, have players use the device once per event, and cross your fingers that such a proposal will happen ...

I've not been in the vans of late, but imagine the situation has not improved. The recent love affair with functional training, led by the influence of the TPI program, has all but destroyed the value of individual exercise machines and the need to isolate muscle function (especially in the case of the lumbar spine). And what has been learned in the process? Nothing - and it wouldn't matter anyway. The latest version of the Cybex Eagle back machine comes with *no* seat belt. They don't know, and I don't think they care.

On a recent tour of neighboring country-club facilities to select equipment for our new fitness center (under construction at the time), I asked the sales representative, *"Why does Cybex (or any manufacturer for that matter) not incorporate the method MedX uses to lift their weight stacks? The patents have expired and the reduced friction would be significant to the longevity of the machines."*

His reply, *"Because there is no demand in the marketplace."*

"No demand for quality?" I asked.

"No ... no demand for machines."

While the quality of what is offered may influence demand, today's physical training for golf (dominated by functional exercise and the TPI program) is driven by a *hands on* approach - the need to have a trainer - which has not gone unnoticed ...

Last winter at a driving range in North Palm Beach, Florida, I conversed with a sales representative for a company that makes a versatile stretching web. He told me that he sold a unit to all three tour vans and heard nothing but positive feedback from the staff of therapists and trainers in follow-up visits. Through the grapevine, however, it was rumored that none of the trainers actually used the device because it threatened their employment. They preferred to stretch clients *by hand* - similar to the medical community's response to the MedX device. I'd love to see the result of a *hand-strengthened* low back.

As far as the lumbar spine is concerned, the finest golfers in the world are victims of general ignorance, lousy equipment, a reluctance to provide the best, and politics.

Let's take a closer look at the muscles of the core.

Low-Back Muscles

The only device shown to isolate, meaningfully access and strengthen the muscles that extend the spine is the MedX® Lumbar Extension machine. If you believe otherwise, review the following:

- Dr. Michael Fulton, Arthur Jones' longtime corporate orthopedic representative, provided medical input during the development of the MedX machine and wrote the following:

    "During the last four years, carefully conducted and large-scale research has clearly proven that less than two minutes of weekly exercise is all that is required in order to strengthen these muscles to a degree that I would not have believed possible as recently as four years ago. Working with this new equipment, using five of our research staff as our first subjects in order to learn what to expect from later and much-larger-scale research, the results were as follows:

    SUBJECT ONE, an increase in the strength of the fully-extended lumbar extension muscles of 180 percent as a result of ten exercises performed over a period of ten weeks. One brief exercise each week.

    SUBJECT TWO, an increase of 450 percent as a result of one exercise every fourteen days for a period of five months.

    SUBJECT THREE, an increase of 877 percent as a result of one exercise performed approximately every fourteen days for a period of twenty-seven weeks.

    SUBJECT FOUR, an increase of 1,460 percent as a result of one exercise every fourteen days for a period of eleven weeks.

    SUBJECT FIVE, an increase of 7,300 percent as a result of one exercise every fourteen days for a period of five months.

    Impossible? I would have said so myself as recently as four years ago, but, as it happens, the last listed of the above five subjects was me.

When first tested, my strength six degrees short of full extension of the lumbar spine produced an output of only four foot-pounds of torque; five months later, in the same position, I produced 296 foot-pounds of torque with the totally isolated muscles that extend the lumbar spine.

To say that we were surprised by the results is to put it mildly indeed, we were stunned.

It is also interesting to note that four out of the above five subjects had been using a Nautilus Lower-back Machine on a regular basis for periods varying from two to six years prior to the start of this isolated exercise."[3]

- The original Nautilus Lower-back machine had a 250-pound weight stack that no one was able to lift during seven years in my gym - but heavy is relative. Subject Four (above) was MedX general manager, Jim Flanagan who *could* lift the entire stack. To accommodate his strength, Jones built a machine with a 450-pound weight stack that, in time, proved equally inadequate. Flanagan routinely performed the exercise, in good form, with two, two-hundred-pound men standing on the weight stack – a total of approximately 850 pounds. Everyone assumed that Jim's initial test on the MedX Lumbar Extension machine was exceptional, but no one was certain because an ideal strength curve and strength norms had not been established. The surprise came when Jim re-tested at eleven weeks, having used the new device briefly only one time every two weeks. He was fifteen times stronger, not 15 percent. The 1,460 percent strength increase in full extension demonstrated one thing – muscle atrophy, the state of his lumbar extensor muscles entering the experiment. Jim could lift 850 pounds on the Nautilus machine, but was *not* strong when his hip muscles were removed from the effort. Strong somewhere - but not where we thought.
- I played golf in Venezuela with a low-back orthopedic specialist/20-year bodybuilder who had a long history of performing weighted hyperextensions off the end of a bench. When my MedX machine arrived in Caracas, I invited the doctor to test his strength. He removed his tie, expanded his chest a few times and, judging by the

color of his face, put forth a noble effort. The results said otherwise. His strength was 20 percent below norms for men his size and age. Years of traditional low-back exercise had not produced the expected result.

- Steve Z. entered my MedX facility in Coral Springs, Florida and introduced himself as the current world-record holder in weightlifting. The size of his hamstrings and butt supported the claim. Steve's intent was to try *"the machine that measured back strength,"* and mentioned a pending competition. The test revealed that he was not *the strongest man in the world.* His low-back strength was slightly below average compared to research norms, and the muscles that produced that result fatigued quickly. The ideal protocol for his fiber-type (established by research) was one minute of exercise every two weeks. Steve knew physiology and insisted on more. He came in once a week until a re-evaluation at four weeks revealed an 18-percent loss in strength - his muscles couldn't tolerate the frequency. From then on, Steve exercised once every two weeks as recommended. A follow-up test revealed that he had not only re-gained the lost strength, but added another 20 percent. Three things were apparent: A career of competitive weightlifting had little to no effect on the strength of his lumbar muscles; brief, infrequent and specific exercise is required to stimulate the muscles of the spine; and, the right tool is required.

- James Graves, PhD conducted MedX Lumbar Extension research at the University of Florida in the late 1980's and early 1990's. When tested for his fatigue characteristics, Graves performed so many repetitions that Jones accused him of not cooperating on the test that determined the selected resistance – but Arthur was wrong. During every test that followed, Graves displayed unparalleled endurance. Immediately after *every* performance, he demonstrated an *increase* in strength. Dr. Graves transferred to Syracuse University where he continued his research. In 1994, he tested the isolated low-back strength of sixteen elite male rowers from the collegiate team and compared the results to norms of untrained men the same size, age and weight (6'2", 190 pounds). According to Graves, the rowers were *"marginally higher at full extension, but not statistically significant. Rowing,"* he concluded, *"does not develop a significant amount of lumbar extension strength."*[4] Why? The motion allows the pelvis to rotate.

- Scott Leggett, a member of Jones' staff, took a series of fatigue tests on the MedX Lumbar Extension machine that revealed a consistent loss of 18 percent strength on pre- and post-exercise tests. On a later occasion during a fatigue test, he performed the exercise to exhaustion using a Nautilus Lower-back machine. The post-exercise test revealed an average increase in strength of 2.5 percent throughout the range of motion, with the exception of a slight decline in full extension. Eleven repetitions to muscle failure on the Nautilus machine had *no* effect on the status of his isolated lumbar extensors (measured by the MedX device), clearly demonstrating the use of *other* muscles during exercise on the Nautilus machine. (Figures 3 and 4, Hole #11)

- Gary Reinl volunteered for a MedX low-back test during *The Challenge of the Lumbar Spine* in New York City (1987), Jones' formal introduction of the new tool. The test revealed an abnormal strength curve, a high rate of fatigue and poor recovery ability (typical of subjects with a predominance of fast-twitch muscle fibers). He decided to do something about it and promptly initiated a three-times-per-week program of exercise on a Cybex Low-back machine. A supposed stronger Reinl re-tested on the MedX machine four years later only to find that he had lost 22 percent of his strength. More motivated, Gary trained for a year on a Nautilus Lower-back machine and, when re-tested on the MedX device, demonstrated the same values. He then worked out a full year on a second-generation Nautilus Lower-back machine only to find that he had further deteriorated. Despite progressively heavier weights on each machine, an awareness of his needs, motivation and plenty of hard work, the muscles that extended his spine *lost* strength for six years. Why? They were never stimulated. Traditional low-back exercise strengthens hip and rear-thigh muscles, but does *not* affect the muscles that extend the spine. *"So far,"* claimed Arthur Jones, *"we have found only two exceptions to that general rule: ONE, so-called 'hyper-extension' movements performed on a simple bench called a 'Roman Chair', and TWO, water-ski activities; but, in both cases, any resulting increases in lower-back strength are produced only near the fully-extended position of the movement."*[5]

When it comes to full-range lumbar extension strength, bodybuilding exercises don't cut it (ask the Venezuelan doctor), typical low-back gym machines don't do it (ask Gary Reinl and Jim Flanagan) and sports activities don't work (ask Steve Z. and the collegiate crew at Syracuse University). And, to no one's surprise - unless you subscribe to functional training - draping a client over a Swiss ball will also, *not* do it.

The most important third of the *core* is clear: *Try as you may, you cannot strengthen the muscles that extend the lumbar spine through traditional means.*

Abdominal Muscles

Functional and sport-specific advocates believe that abdominal muscles are vital to performance, while the medical community touts their contribution to low-back rehabilitation and muscle balance. The stance, they believe, has been proven by research and by thousands of successful medical applications. Its popularity has resulted in a surge of gym activity – trainees dedicating as much time to minor muscle groups as major, and the exclusive use of functional tools (or none at all) to strengthen the abdomen.

The Nautilus inventor had a different take. When Arthur Jones successfully trained Casey Viator for the Mr. America title in 1971, he let the abdomen *take care of itself* - and it did. No exercise for the abdomen for eleven months before the contest led to abs that favorably compared to the best in the history of the sport. Following a decade of prodding, Jones developed an abdominal machine to complete his Nautilus line; but he failed to include any such device among his MedX testing and rehabilitation tools. Was the challenge too great? I think not. The PhD's at the University of Florida called Jones *"a genius in body mechanics and exercise physiology."* He was thorough and honest. If he perceived a value - *any* value - of abdominal strength to corporal stimulation, athletic performance or to the treatment of chronic back pain, he would have declared so on the spot, and addressed the problem. But the abdomen did not grab his attention – which makes today's frenzy more suspicious.

Following two back surgeries, I have not performed *any* abdominal exercise for thirty-five years. If I chose to resume the exercises I performed *before* the surgeries, I would ignore today's *core* offerings and select something more efficient and effective – like the best abdominal tool available. And it goes without saying, if I had a bicycle and a Bentley in my garage, I would not insist on riding the bike.

My low back is as strong as I can make it (through MedX Lumbar exercise) but my abdomen is not - a fact of great concern to those who believe in muscle balance. Could I feel better, or perform better, by working abdominal muscles? Perhaps … but I'll never know. I prefer to prove a lot of people wrong.

Oblique Muscles

The core is flanked by muscles on each side called *obliques* that laterally bend and rotate the torso. This endears them to many sports - including golf - and to current trends in exercise, where their importance depends upon whom you ask. Jones recognized the value of strong oblique muscles in the treatment of chronic low-back pain and spent fourteen years developing a medical rotary-torso machine for that purpose.

Typically, torso-rotation machines in gyms are among the most abused. Jones built several models that restricted hip movement while the upper-body rotated, but was never satisfied with the degree of muscle isolation provided. He later unveiled a prototype that fixed the upper body and allowed the lower body to rotate, but it was never marketed. In the end, there was no discussion about the isolation provided by his medical device, or of proper use. It's tough to talk when you can barely breathe.

Modern oblique training generally takes a simple core exercise and adds a twist, which provides unlimited variety – nothing more. Dr. Fulton once witnessed a physical therapist attach a latex resistance band to the frame of a $60,000 MedX Torso Rotation machine to perform a standing version of the same. *"Like tying a horse to your car,"* he commented, *"and pulling it around town."*

To the therapist's credit, it was state-of-the-art tubing.

Trainees are often brainwashed by functional trainers who rarely choose the most efficient or effective path. Don't mess around: Find the best tool and get the job done.

Muscle Balance

Most *core* advocates believe - as the medical community before - that spinal muscles are stronger than abdominal muscles, despite a decade of research at the University of Florida that clearly demonstrates the contrary.

Balanced development is important for joint stability, but how is it defined? How would you know if and when you were balanced? MedX research[6] has established an *ideal* strength curve for the isolated muscles that extend the lumbar spine through a full range of motion, but the same has not been established for abdominal muscles. Without proper equipment, the only option is to strengthen muscles on all sides of a joint with tools that change the resistance according to the ideal strength curve of each muscle through a complete range of motion. That means use of machines with a proper cam or lever system – pure heresy for core experts who prefer exercises that fail to provide full-range strength, including static postures which limit gains to a few angles. And then they claim, *"If you feel better, you just might be balanced."* A monkey can do better than that.

Another point: Judging from the poor strength levels of the majority of low backs in this country, it would be hard to imagine abdominal muscles as worse. Which means: Those who initiate *core* training probably have an abdomen stronger than low back - *without* knowing. And, because it is *not* possible to strengthen low-back muscles through traditional means, any attempt to strengthen the core - both front and back - results in the strengthening of abdominals only, which makes the initial imbalance worse.

I rest my case.

General Balance

The introduction of core exercise to the fitness industry was accompanied by a related entity – balance training. The connection was clear: Establishing or maintaining balance activates muscles of the core, and it didn't take long to appear in golf performance programs. The glaring difference in balance between amateurs and professionals, between good and bad players, and the diminished balance that accompanies the aging process made it an easy sell.

My first exposure to balance training was awkward, but simple: A client voiced the request, and I fetched the equipment. I survived the session without knowing a thing about it and headed for the library. What I learned was this: Balance is an underlying *ability* that supports a skill, is genetically determined at an early age (about 5-6 years), and is not subject to change[7], meaning it can't be trained. I should have issued a refund.

The perceptible improvement in balance experienced in the practice of a task performed on a gym floor can be attributed to an improvement in skill - a skill in which balance plays a prominent underlying role. As skill improves, so does balance – but ONLY in reference to that skill. Balance does NOT transfer from one skill to another, which makes the ridiculous combinations of balance, skill and strength in the TPI program more absurd. To stand on an unstable apparatus while you throw and receive a weighted ball in a golf swing motion, for example, is useless to everyone but the instructor. He or she can rationalize the activity by spouting phrases such as *power, acceleration, balance* and *just like your backswing*. But the truth is - from the perspective of skill or balance - *just like* doesn't cut it.

Balance is important to golf but, plain and simple, it cannot be improved by practicing a related skill that features the element of balance in an exercise setting. The application must be specific: The next time you frequent the practice tee, try to hit *every* shot with *perfect* balance, and pose at the end of *every* swing. That will improve your bottom line more than anything you can accomplish in a gym.

Conclusion

The importance of core training to golf can be put into perspective by looking at the many tour professionals who do not perform core exercise, or any exercise at all. Would they be more effective if they were fit? Yes, but many are competitive *as is,* and content to remain so.

I'm not opposed to strengthening any muscle: Doing so would improve performance if that muscle is involved in the activity. What I object to is the emphasis on *core* muscles at the expense of those that create a greater ripple in the pond. And, I'm not a fan of poor equipment, when better is available.

If you insist on strengthening *core* muscles: Perform one set of 8-12 repetitions on a MedX Lumbar Extension machine (once a week); and one set of 8-12 repetitions on the best torso-rotation and abdominal machines you can find (twice a week). The five-minute total will create time for what you'd rather do – hone your golf skills.

Truth has a way of evading the field of exercise, and core training is no exception.

Let's examine, in greater detail, the muscles that extend the lumbar spine and a proven means to strengthen them.

References

1. Marguerite Ogle, "Core Strength," *pilates.about*, November (2014), http://www.pilates.about.com/od/pilatesterms/g/CoreStrength.htm
2. James Graves et al., "Pelvic Stabilization During Resistance Training: Its Effect on the Development of Lumbar Extension Strength," *Archives of Physical Medicine and Rehabilitation* 75 (1994), 210.
3. Michael Fulton, "Lower-Back Pain: a New Solution For An Old Problem," MedX Corporation publication (1988).
4. S.F. Szuba et al., "Effect of Lumbar Extension Training in Collegiate Rowers," *Medicine and Science in Sports and Exercise* 27 (1995), S21.
5. Arthur Jones, "The Future of Exercise: 1997 and Beyond," *arthurjonesexercise*, http://www.arthurjonesexercise.com./Future_Exercise/6.PDF
6. James Graves et al., "Quantitative Assessment of Full Range-of-Motion Isometric Lumbar Extension Strength," *Spine* 15 (1990), 289.
7. Brian Johnston, *System Analysis* (Sudbury, ON: Bodyworx Publishing, 2001), 137.

Hole #11: 195 Yards, Par 3

THE LOW-BACK HOAX

On a pitch-black Monday morning in 1974, I followed a hasty breakfast with a trip to Lookout Point where, at the crack of dawn, I would warm up before the drive to Lewiston, NY. The Niagara Falls Country Club, site of the Porter Cup qualifier, was more than an hour away. My tee time was early; and my timing, perfect. The moment I could see, I began my routine – a few stretching movements, wedge shots, nine-iron, then eight and down the line – just as I had hundreds of times. I was playing well and believed I could qualify, as I had the year before.

Things went smoothly until a swing with a driver shot a bolt of pain down my left leg. I hobbled to the car hoping to feel better at the other end. Not so. Plan B - aim left and cross your fingers – and the brevity of my follow-through won a friendly wave from the security guard at the exit.

Anyone who has played the game has probably experienced something similar. Rotation of the body, impact with ball and turf, and the strain of extension in the follow-through can all contribute to back issues. Yet, high forces applied to the body during the swing are only half the story. Injury to spinal muscles is more likely caused by rapid acceleration, or rapid deceleration. The club-head speed of the average PGA Tour professional is 115-120 miles per hour (with a driver). At address, or in a balanced finish position, the speed is zero. The safety of that scenario can only be countered by strong muscles, or advanced skill.

The skill aspect is often addressed, but the strength element remains ignored.

In his first on-course interview following back surgery, Tiger Woods claimed he was bored performing all the little exercises for his back (those common to the rehab process; exercises that have their time and place). He talked about strengthening abdominal and glute muscles, but not a word about his low back. According to Arthur Jones, strong abdominal muscles have *nothing* to do with back pain, and strong butt muscles are often the cause of back problems. The *little exercises* for Tiger's back might serve to relieve symptoms, but they fail to fully prepare him for the demands of the game. According to a decade of research at the University of Florida and the University of California at San Diego, traditional exercises performed for the purpose of strengthening the muscles that extend the lumbar spine have no effect. Why? The pelvis is allowed to rotate during back extension movements.

The only tool known to effectively prevent such rotation during exercise is the MedX Lumbar Extension machine. Unfortunately, the only thing that prevents a touring pro's pelvis from rotating are therapists and trainers who don't believe in machines, or in *seated* exercise; and those wed to companies that falsely claim their equipment *strengthens* the lumbar spine.

That's where the Nautilus inventor stepped in.

In January of 1972, Arthur Jones announced to a handful of employees, *"I plan to build a machine that totally isolates muscle function. When I say something about a muscle, it will be 100 percent of that muscle, nothing less. The machine will take approximately six months to build at a cost of $200,000."* Deep down, he believed he could complete the task in three weeks for less than ten thousand dollars.

To add to the challenge, Jones selected the muscles of the front thigh (quadriceps); and later, those that extend the lumbar spine (erector spinae).

He began by modifying existing tools to test the strength of front and rear thighs, but the process took more than a few weeks. *"An acceptable version of such a machine,"* he said, *"was not produced until April of 1991, nineteen years and three months after we started. Even a few months earlier, and after years of continuous work, it still appeared to be an impossible undertaking; every time we solved one problem we became aware of other, previously unsuspected problems."*

The challenge to develop a tool to isolate the lumbar extensor muscles was equally complex. Jones first applied a variable resistance to the working muscles by having trainees push a large, round pad applied to the upper back as it extended through a full range-of-motion from a seated position. The result: The Nautilus Lower-back machine became the first tool to provide *direct* exercise for the muscles of the spine. He then attached a strain gauge to the device to examine the relationship between muscle strength and low-back pain. It led to a shocking conclusion: The device didn't work.

> *When I designed that machine, I clearly understood that it provided exercise for both the hip and thigh muscles ... but I believed that it also provided meaningful exercise for the lumbar-extensor muscles; an assumption that I now realize was wrong. The machine is misnamed, is in fact a hip and thigh machine, provides meaningful exercise only for the muscles of the buttocks and rear of the thighs.*[1]

In simple terms, the machine allowed the pelvis to rotate, which activated the large muscles of the hip. It also activated his competitors. Following decades of research that supported Jones' contention, every major exercise-machine manufacturer copied - *and continues to copy* - a back machine that he warned, "...*will do nothing for the strength of lower-back muscles.*"

Jones continued his quest and successfully anchored the pelvis in a 'stand-up' model. *"The pelvis did* not *rotate,"* he claimed, *"but it took two people to put you in, and three to drag you out."*

The final solution struck like lightning: Use the femur (the upper-thigh bone that attaches to the pelvis) to *indirectly* prevent pelvic rotation. Illustrated below (Figure 1), Jones wedged the femur into the pelvis at an angle controlled by a small pad located above the knee. The force generated by a crank that moved the foot platform (A) toward the hips (in the direction of the arrows) prevented the pelvis from moving forward. The thigh-restraint belt (B) simultaneously provided a fulcrum to control the angle at which the femur contacted the pelvis and to prevent the pelvis from rising during extension. Properly secured, the pelvis could not move forward, and no longer rise. The problem appeared solved, but for Jones. *"Believing that the pelvis is not moving during testing or exercise is not good enough,"* he said. *"You must* know *that the pelvis is not moving."* Proof was ultimately provided by a round, free-moving pad placed behind the pelvis (C). If the pelvis rotated one millimeter, the pad moved two - and any undesired movement could be eliminated by tightening the footboard and/ or thigh-restraint mechanism. The significance of the degree of stability provided by the new device was yet to be determined.

Figure 1: **Muscle Isolation - Pelvic Restraint**

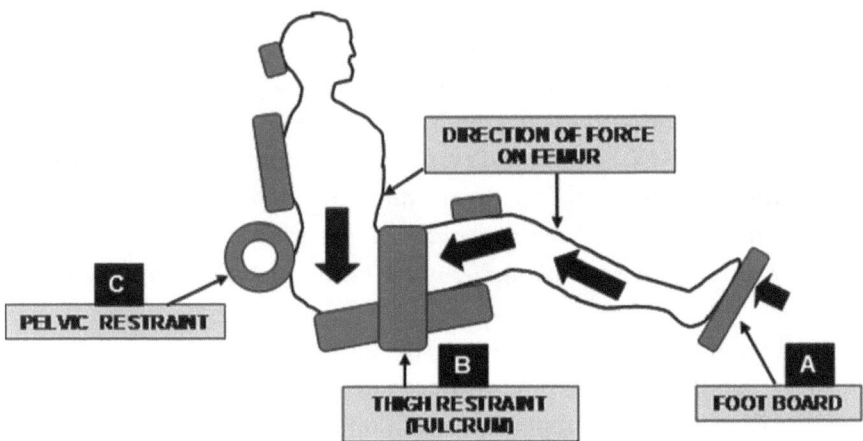

Fourteen years, three thousand prototypes and eighty-eight million dollars later, Jones introduced the MedX Lumbar Extension machine at *The Challenge of the Lumbar Spine* in the Waldorf Astoria Hotel, New York City, October 8th and 9th, 1987. To advertize the event, he published a full-page article in *The Washington Post*, titled, *A Partial Solution for a Forty-Billion-Dollar Annual Problem for Industry, Insurance and Government – Screening for Lower Back Problems*. The statistical evidence from ten thousand lumbar evaluations identified three risk factors associated with the incidence of low-back problems: *One*, Muscle Fiber-Type; *Two*, 'Specific' or 'General' Response to Exercise; and *Three*, Chronic Disuse Atrophy.

One: Muscle fiber-type relates to the rate of muscle fatigue, a genetic factor. Some low-back muscles possess an abundance of *fast-twitch* fibers that are stronger than average and capable of producing explosive power, but they fatigue quickly with repetitive use. Other low-back muscles possess an abundance of *slow-twitch* fibers that are weaker, better suited to repetitive tasks (endurance), and less likely to suffer low-back problems.

Two: A 'Specific' response to exercise occurs when a muscle fatigues (short-term) or grows (long-term) *only within* the range of motion that it performs exercise. A 'General' response to exercise occurs when a muscle fatigues or grows *throughout* the range of motion, regardless of the range in which work is performed. A muscle with a 'General' response is less likely to encounter back problems.

Three: Infrequent use of the MedX Lumbar Extension machine results in dramatic and rapid strength increases in approximately 90 percent of subjects following a twelve-week protocol. The magnitude of increase indicates a widespread prevalence of muscle atrophy.

Figure 2 (below) illustrates the three risk factors associated with the muscles that extend the lumbar spine, and provides insight into the fact that approximately 80 percent of people suffer back pain.

Figure 2: **Risk Factors For Spinal Injury**

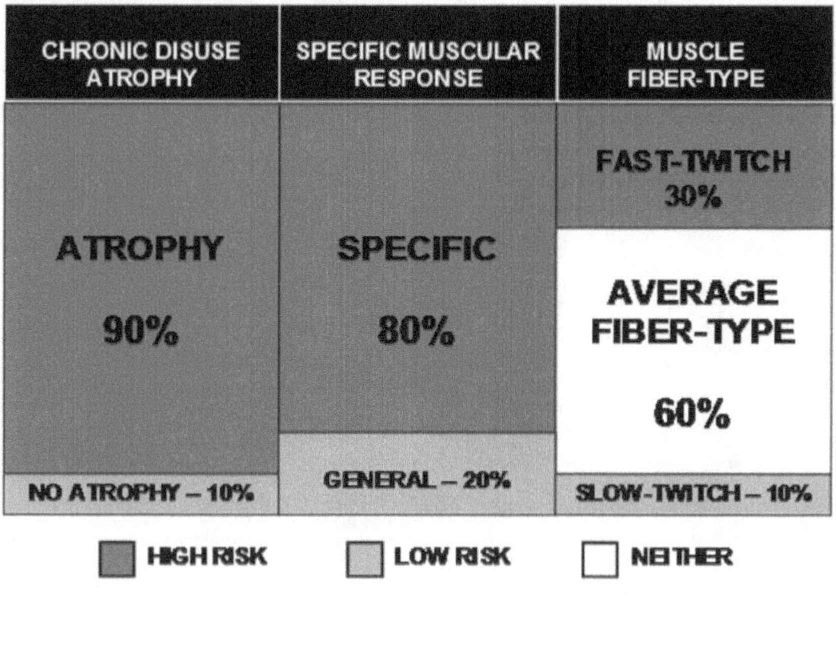

The Right Tool

Jones first tested the isolated low-back strength of five staff members who had used his Nautilus Lower-back machine for years, exposed them to an exercise protocol and retested their strength. He was surprised to find an *explosion* in strength (as if they had done *no* prior exercise). It was clear that pelvic restraint truly isolated - and exercised - a different set of muscles. To further demonstrate, Jones subjected one of the five subjects to a series of muscle-fatigue tests: a pre-exercise test of fresh strength, followed *immediately* by a challenging exercise to muscle failure, and *immediately* by a post-exercise test of exhausted strength. The difference between pre- and post-exercise values revealed the short-term effect of the exercise. The results of one such test are illustrated below.

Figure 3 demonstrates strength loss from a pre- (#1) and post- (#2) exercise test. When the subject performed exhausting exercise on a device that prevented pelvic rotation (MedX), he consistently lost 18-20 percent of his strength due to fatigue (a value confirmed by similar evaluations).

Figure 4 demonstrates the same pre- (#1) and post- (#2) muscle-fatigue tests with one difference: Exercise - between the tests – was performed on a Nautilus Lower back machine. This time, there was *no* strength loss when exercise was performed *with* pelvic rotation (Nautilus), which means that lumbar extensor muscles *were not used* when the pelvis was allowed to rotate.

Figure 3:

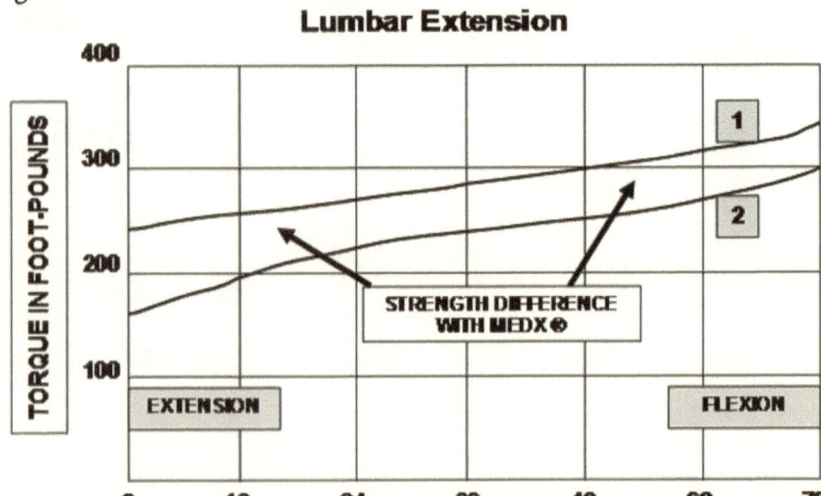

122

Figure 4:

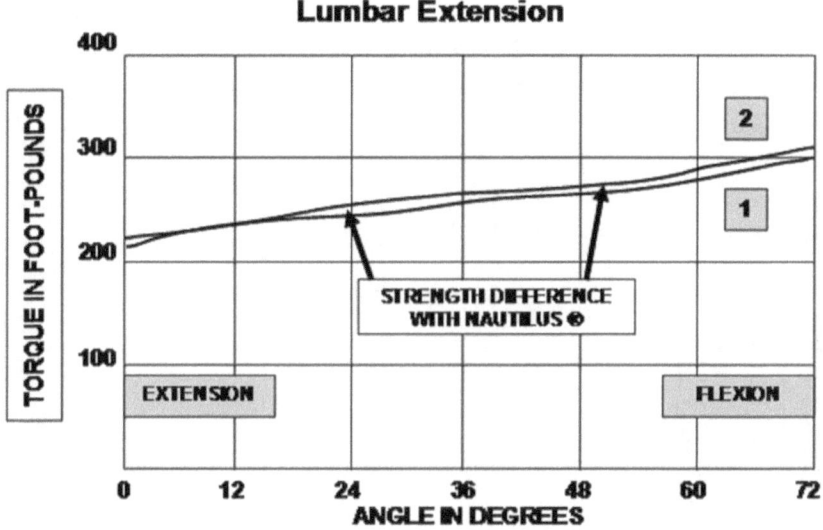

It was clear: Traditional low-back exercise that allows pelvic rotation works the large muscles of the hip. The small muscles that extend the back *do not contribute to, nor benefit from* the effort.

Official Confirmation

To verify the effectiveness of his new device, Jones established the Center for Exercise Science at the University of Florida in Gainesville, where initial studies focused on the accuracy and reliability of the MedX Lumbar Extension machine, the establishment of an effective exercise protocol and the need for pelvic stability during exercise.

Figure 5 (below) represents a research study[2] that determined the training effect of commercial low-back machines on the development of isolated lumbar-extension strength. Seventy-seven healthy subjects tested their strength on a MedX Lumbar Extension machine and were randomly divided into four groups. One group trained on the Nautilus Lower-back machine; one on the Cybex Eagle Low-back machine; one on the MedX machine; and one not at all (Control Group; Curve #2). All groups performed one exercise per week for twelve weeks and re-tested their strength on the MedX device.

The results follow:

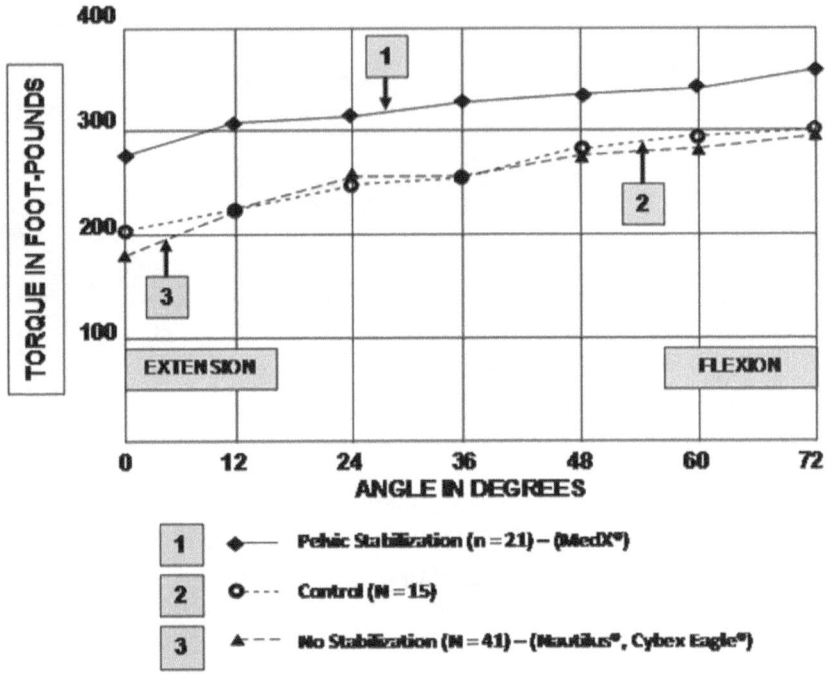

Figure 5: **The Effect Of Training With Pelvic Stabilization On Lumbar Extension Strength**

Both Nautilus and Cybex Eagle groups showed no change in isolated lumbar extension strength at any of the measured angles. Their results were combined into a *No Stabilization* group (Curve #3) for comparative purposes. The MedX group (Curve #1) showed a significant increase in isometric strength at each angle throughout the range of motion. An interesting observation in the study was the increase in dynamic strength (the amount of weight lifted) in *all* groups – proof that the added resistance was being lifted by *other* muscles.

The implications are clear: *One*, pelvic stabilization is necessary to elicit a training effect in the muscles that extend the spine; and *Two*, the stabilization provided by commercial back machines is inadequate.

The next step was to investigate the effect of strength on chronic pain. This involved introduction of the device to a medical community that already believed a high percentage of back problems were muscular (or soft tissue) in nature - a perfect fit. *"Damage to the soft tissue in the region of the lumbar spine"*, claimed Jones, *"will seldom be revealed by an X-ray, may or may not be detected by a CAT-scan or by Magnetic Resonance Imaging ... but almost certainly will be discovered by this test."*

Jones established a second education/research site at the University of California, San Diego, under the direction of renowned orthopedic, Dr. Vert Mooney. At its peak, the center treated eight hundred people per week to a twelve-week lumbar protocol. The volume of statistics hastened a conclusion concerning the effect of isolated exercise on chronic back pain. *"If you have been suggested for low-back surgery,"* declared Dr. Mooney, *"you would be crazy not to try the MedX Lumbar Extension machine as a last resort."*

Not only did the MedX machine target the desired muscles through proper stabilization, it forced trainees to adopt proportionate strength at every angle of movement by delivering the correct resistance to the muscles through a full range-of-motion. It was long overdue:

> *The magnitude of gain shown by the training group reflects the low initial trained strength of the lumbar extensor muscles. These data indicate that when the lumbar area is isolated through pelvic stabilization, the isolated lumbar extensor muscles show an abnormally large potential for strength increase.* [3] (in this study, a 102 percent increase in extension and 42 percent increase in flexion)

Figure 6 (below) demonstrates the collective results produced by the first group of subjects to use the Medx device for prolonged exercise. The grey columns (left side at each angle) represent the average static strength of the isolated back muscles measured *before* an exercise protocol that lasted from ten to twenty-seven weeks. The black columns (right side at each angle) represent strength levels *after* the protocol. All subjects had a two-to-six-year history on the Nautilus Lower-back machine.

Figure 6: **Strength Gains**

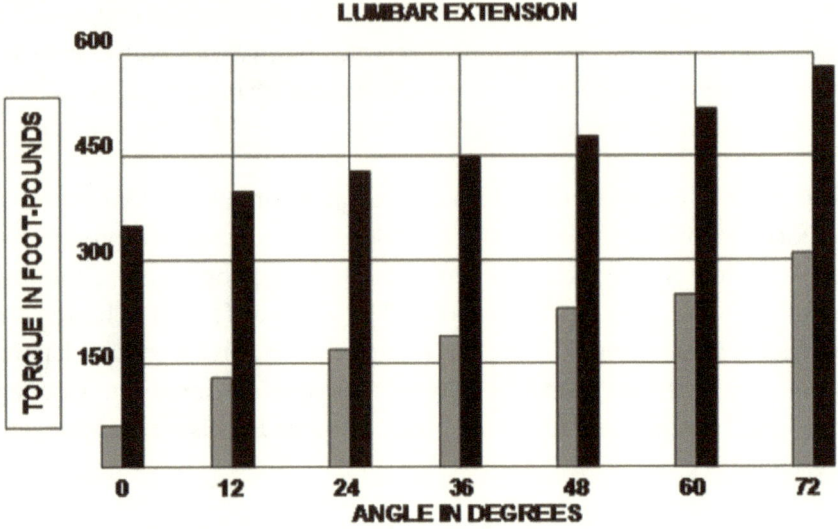

The average increase in the level of peak torque (strength) in flexion (right side of chart) was 87 percent, while the average in extension (left side) was 686 percent. The average overall strength increase throughout the range of motion was 142 percent.

The dramatic result required little exercise. The MedX machine was used, at most, once a week and, at least, once every two weeks; and the average time per exercise was less than two minutes. The official protocol in a clinical setting was established: Twice a week for the first month; once a week for the next two months.

The protocol for strength maintenance was equally simple and effective:

> *These findings indicate that isometric lumbar extension strength can be maintained for up to twelve weeks with a reduced frequency of training as low as once every four weeks when the intensity and the volume of exercise are maintained.* [4]

Figure 7 (below) illustrates the staying power of specific exercise for the lumbar spine. The black columns (right side at each angle) represent the average strength level of a large group of subjects following a twelve-week program of exercise on the MedX machine. The grey columns (left side at each angle) represent isometric strength following an additional twelve weeks of training using a frequency of one exercise every four weeks - no change in the first half of the range of motion (right side of chart); a one percent increase at mid-range; and a seven percent decrease in extension (left side of chart). Having increased the strength of the spinal muscles with specific exercise, very little in the way of additional exercise is required to maintain a peak level of strength.

Figure 7: **Strength Maintenance**

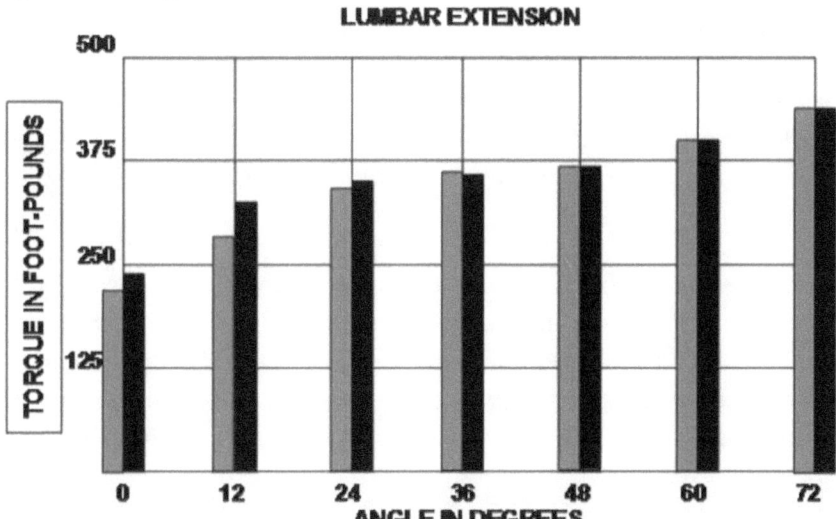

The conclusions of the studies represented by Figures 6 and 7 (*above*) indicate the following:

1. Lumbar extensor muscles are generally in an atrophied state.
2. Low-frequency training is effective for increasing the strength of the muscles that extend the lumbar spine, in contrast to what is shown when training other muscle groups.
3. Lumbar-extension strength increases occur mainly within the first twelve weeks of training, although additional gains in the extended positions can be expected when training is continued through twenty weeks.
4. Changes in peak strength are not indicative of changes throughout the lumbar extensor range-of-motion.

5. The muscles that extend the lumbar spine are unique in their response to exercise. They do *not* require much to attain peak strength, and very little to maintain.

When all clinical research was on the table, 80 percent of patients with chronic back pain (regardless of diagnosis) reported a reduction in pain perception after a twelve-week MedX protocol. Thirty to thirty-three percent became pain free. The success of the treatment prompted Arthur Jones to state toward the end of his career: *"If and when the government ever takes any meaningful steps in the direction of sanity, which I doubt, it could come to pass that all cases of lower-back pain will be treated first with MedX machines, that any other treatment will be prohibited until and unless MedX treatment has been tried and has failed. A simple federal law to that effect would save the people in this country a minimum of $80,000,000,000.00 a year."*[5]

Despite the success of the MedX tool, most trainers are unaware of its existence, or continue to ignore the facts. In the meantime, the powers-to-be have all but destroyed the value of muscle isolation, discredited the use of machines in general, ignored everything related to the work of Arthur Jones and replaced it with a ten-cent solution - a Swiss Ball and bodyweight exercise.

Its lack of recognition extends beyond the scope of exercise. *"MedX spinal therapy has amassed impressive research results,"* claims one research scientist, *"but little name recognition."* Research publications typically mention the manufacturer's name once and often fail to identify what really produced the result.

And the press has not helped. In a *New York Times* report on Dr. Brian Nelson's study (above), MedX therapy was identified as *weight lifting*. When *weight lifting* is deemed effective in the treatment of chronic back pain, images of exercises that likely add to the problem, vault to the fore.

The ultimate insult was delivered by the medical community: MedX treatment was perceived a threat. Dr. Nelson co-authored a review of literature published in the January edition of *Medicine and Science in Sports and Exercise,* 1999, that represented an historical perspective of exercise related to spine care. *"Strengthening exercises,"* he stated, *"were initially used for physical therapy rather than general conditioning."* Somewhere down the line things changed. *"A review of 'modern' spine care over the past thirty years shows that these early concepts were abandoned in favor of passive modalities that predominantly treat symptoms."*[6] To this day, the efficacy of passive modalities lacks scientific evidence; the efficacy of MedX treatment does not.

The MedX Lumbar Extension machine provides the *only* means to meaningfully access and strengthen the muscles that extend the lumbar spine. And for one reason: The machine does *not* allow the pelvis to rotate during exercise.

Its twelve-week protocol, properly performed, can achieve the following:

- Increase functional range of motion.
- Establish proportionate and full-range strength.
- Modify strength curves to approximate the *ideal*.
- Reduce or eliminate pain perception in chronic cases.
- Address the root cause of the majority of low-back problems – lack of muscle strength.

Conclusion

The story that follows, provided by USMA Hall-of-Fame football legend, Dick Nowak, illustrates the need for the proper tool:

> *In the fall of 1957, senior center Paul Barre took the field for the Bartlett High School varsity football team in Webster, Massachusetts in what would be no ordinary contest. The Indians hosted arch-rival Putnam High – both, undefeated.*
>
> *Paul was prepared. He had practiced all week with star-quarterback, Joseph White III, who had earned the title, The Magician for pulling out a game earlier in the schedule. In fact, as the season progressed, Joseph believed he was the go-to guy who could pull out any game.*

This one came down to the wire. With less than two minutes to play in a scoreless battle, Bartlett blocked a field-goal attempt and got the ball back.

The re-energized quarterback rallied his troops in the huddle and called a play. In the anxiety of the moment, the team got the snap count wrong and jumped offside. The ball never moved. Back in the huddle, White made it clear, "You know I'm a magician, but I need the ball."

The formidable wall of green and white lined up a second time. Bob Sellig dug his cleats into the turf. Paul Barre re-established his stance. Dick Nowak was primed to go. But Joseph White III was not. He didn't like what he saw, and checked off the play at scrimmage.

Paul was his vocal self, "Are you kidding me?"

The reply from above was swift, "No."

Paul quickly turned his head toward his line-mates and hollered, "He's pulling another one out of his hat – The Magician."

The team's laughter shattered the seriousness of the moment. The game ended in a 0-0 tie.*

> **Dick Nowak captained Army's football team in 1963 and achieved All-American status for his two-way contributions as offensive guard and defensive linebacker.*

You can't weigh yourself with a toaster. The anti-isolation, anti-machine, anti-seated, anti-anything-of-value TPI program does *not* have the right tool. Joseph White III did not have it; and functional trainers don't have it, and don't seem to get it. And if golfers don't get it, they will likely suffer low-back pain.

No magic here - find the right tool before it's too late.

References

1. Arthur Jones, *The Lumbar Spine* (Santa Barbara, CA: Sequoia Communications, 1988), 36.
2. James Graves et al., "Pelvic Stabilization During Resistance Training: Its Effect on the Development of Lumbar Extension Strength," *Archives of Physical Medicine and Rehabilitation* 75, no. 2 (1994), 210.
3. Michael Pollock et al., "Effect of Resistance Training on Lumbar Extension Strength," *The American Journal of Sports Medicine* 17, no. 5 (1989), 624.
4. Jacqueline Tucci et al., "Effect of Reduced Frequency of Training and Detraining on Lumbar Extension Strength," *Spine* 17, no. 12 (1992).
5. Arthur Jones, "My First Half-Century in the Iron Game," *arthurjonesexercise*, http://www.arthurjonesexercise.com./First_Half/61.PDF
6. David M. Carpenter and Brian Nelson, "Low Back Strengthening for the Prevention and Treatment of Low Back Pain," *Medicine and Science in Sports and Exercise* 31, no. 1 (1999), 18.

Hole #12: 523 Yards, Par 5

FULL-RANGE EXERCISE

His record spoke volumes: four-time Canadian Amateur champion, four invitations to the Masters, eight-time Ontario Amateur champion, six-time Canadian Senior Amateur champion, low amateur in the Canadian Open sixteen times, and a member of seventeen Canadian international amateur teams. It was an honor when Nick 'The Wedge' Weslock, one of the finest golfers to ever play the game, graced your invitational tournament - as he did ours in the late 1960's.

Nick loved the history of the game and the challenge of Lookout Point. I was in my late teens when I was first introduced to *the man who could destroy opponents at will*. I recall a barrel chest, Popeye forearms and an immaculate presence – colorful shirt, checked cap, spit-polished shoes and clubs. Nick Weslock was *class* personified - a gentleman who displayed plenty of grit by walking our hilly layout with two hip replacements, and keeping it under par.

Some have it, and some don't. Nick had it – for a long time.

Two years before I was born, 28 year-old Weslock – recognized as one of the best hot-shot amateurs in the country - played a tournament at the Rockway Golf Club in Kitchener, Ontario. With the event on the line, he stepped to the tee of the par-3 sixteenth and glanced at his caddy.

"This is a seven-iron shot," he said.

"No, it's an eight iron," replied the scruffy seventeen year-old assigned to him by head pro, Lloyd Tucker. The kid was nothing to look at, but had been spot-on all day with club selection.

"You sure?"

"Look, you hit the seven-iron and you'll carry your bag from here in."

Weslock blinked hard, shocked by the response. He hit the eight-iron three feet from the flag, sank the putt and went on to win the tournament.

The caddy assigned to Nick that day was Moe Norman, who knew the course like the back of his hand. The opposites became best friends from that day on.

Success in golf depends on the right tools and sound advice. It's no different with exercise.

My introduction to the term, *full-range exercise* came when I overheard a conversation between Ellington Darden, Ph.D., and a client. *"The value of an exercise,"* claimed Darden, *"is a product of the quality of resistance and the range of motion over which the resistance is effective."* It was a phrase I never forgot. At the time, Darden was Director of Research at Nautilus Sports/Medical Industries and had written more than twenty books related to strength training. The *product* to which he referred was *full-range exercise* – the application of an optimum resistance to the working muscles through a complete range of motion.

To understand the term, let's examine a common exercise that does *not* meet the criteria of full-range exercise – a standing biceps curl performed with a barbell. All free-weight exercises deal with two factors: The weight of the implement and the effect of gravity. When the barbell moves vertically or straight up, the effect of gravity (a straight-down pull) is at its greatest. Any direction other than vertical diminishes the effect of gravity and makes the resistance *feel* lighter.

The straight-line resistance of a free-weight exercise (straight-line meaning the vertical pull of gravity) applied to a rotational joint system is not an ideal fit. You can't negotiate a curve in the road by driving in a straight line.

From the starting position of a biceps curl (A, below), the resistance moves away from the thighs in an arc. The direction of movement is not completely vertical until forearms reach a position parallel to the floor (B). At that angle – and only that angle – the resistance *feels* heaviest. From that point upward, the resistance resumes its arc to a final position near the upper chest (C). The first third of the movement feels easy, the middle third difficult, and the final third easy once again. Is the muscle challenged evenly throughout the movement? No. Is it challenged in a position of full extension (A, at the start of the movement)? No. Is it challenged in a position of full contraction, C, where a higher percentage of muscle fibers can be activated to stimulate strength change? No. Is there any value to the exercise? Yes, a value limited by the tool.

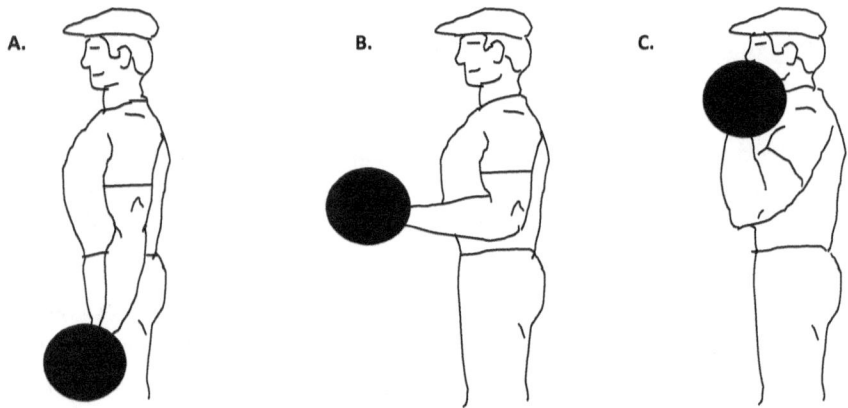

A decade of research at the University of Florida shows that approximately 80 percent of human muscle responds to exercise in a *Specific* manner. That is, muscles fatigue - or gain strength - only within the range of motion where work is performed. In the case of the biceps curl with a barbell, the work zone is represented by the middle third of the exercise. Little work is performed at the beginning of each repetition (near full-extension) or towards the end (near full-contraction). Repetition of such exercise over time results in a strength curve similar to Curve B in Figure 1 (below) – high strength values in the mid-range of motion, lower values elsewhere.

The following chart compares the delivery of resistance provided by a barbell *versus* a Nautilus machine during an upper-arm biceps curl.

Figure 1:

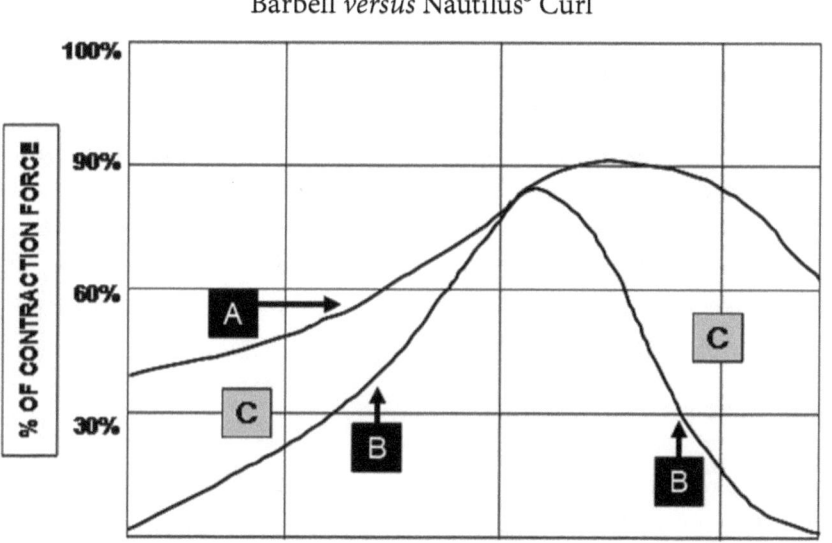

Barbell *versus* Nautilus® Curl

The bottom curve (B) depicts the resistance provided by a barbell. The top curve (A) represents that provided by use of a Nautilus machine (an ideal strength curve determined by force output, and provided by the machine's cam). The area between the curves (C) shows the difference between real and ideal, the additional benefit of a machine that provides a proper distribution of resistance *throughout* the muscle's range of motion.

Figure 1 demonstrates the failure of most free-weight exercises to deliver full-range exercise, and produce full-range strength. The why is clear: The majority of human movement involves rotation around an axis, which produces an arc-like motion. Rotational movement against straight-line gravity produces a *sticking point*, a position that feels difficult to surpass. With few exceptions, sticking points accompany most free-weight and bodyweight exercises.

Full-range exercise occurs when sticking points are eliminated by an exercise cam or leverage system that exposes working muscles to: *One*, an ideal and maximum resistance at *every* angle of movement; and *Two*, a resistance applied at 180 degrees to the muscle's direction of pull. With these criteria in place, an exercise should deliver what feels like an *equal* challenge to working muscles throughout the range of motion.

The quality of resistance and production of full-range strength depends entirely upon choice of tools. If you know nothing about equipment, close your eyes during exercise. If the resistance feels *even* throughout the movement, you have made a good choice. Most free-weight advocates disagree. Their muscles have developed a bias that has led them to believe that the *even* feel provided by a machine is dead wrong - when they are. The *even* feel represents what they choose to ignore - *full-range exercise.*

Equipment

The choice of effective strength-training equipment is far from foolproof, yet one thing is certain. The popular choice of TPI trainers - latex bands, free weights, pulley stations, weighted balls, TRX straps and multi-use machines – may provide an advantage in portability, space or flexibility of use, but they collectively fail to provide the ingredients that satisfy the requirements of full-range exercise. They do *not* provide a consistent muscle challenge, an even feel throughout the execution of an exercise; and do *not* provide the quality or quantity of resistance needed to optimize muscle strength – the only productive factor in performance.

On the other hand, not all exercise machines are perfect or superior. Many are poorly constructed, and fail to deliver a suitable quantitative or qualitative resistance to the working muscles - an *even* feel throughout the movement.

Some machines are probably as good as they'll get. A typical gym leg press, for example, magnifies the selected resistance by three to four times as legs are extended. In other words, a 200-pound resistance could equal eight hundred pounds by the time you extend your legs - which sounds dangerous, but is not. The adjustment provided by a cam or lever system on most leg-press machines fails to challenge the working muscles because the leverage provided by the body's moving parts changes at a quicker rate - making an 800-pound resistance in the final angles of extension feel *easy*. Golfers need not be concerned. Performance programs ignore leg-press machines not because of perceived danger, but because the exercise occurs on a device that does not allow *all boots on the ground*.

Good luck.

The ingredients that satisfy the requirements for full-range exercise were identified by Arthur Jones in 1970, and reported by Dr. Ellington Darden[1] thereafter:

1. *Rotary Form Resistance* - resistance that rotates on a common axis with the body part that is directly moved by the exercised muscle.
2. *Direct Resistance* - the application of resistance directly to the body part being moved by the exercised muscle.
3. *Automatically Variable Resistance* - since leverage and strength vary throughout the range of motion, resistance must vary according to the muscle's needs or its potential strength curve.
4. *Balanced Resistance* - to vary the resistance accurately, the movement arm itself must be counterbalanced to prevent its weight from skewing the outcome.
5. *Positive Work* - the provision of a muscle to lift a weight (produce a concentric contraction).
6. *Negative Work* - the provision of a muscle to lower a weight (produce an eccentric contraction).
7. *Stretching* - the ability to pull a muscle to a position that temporarily exceeds its existing range of motion.
8. *Pre-Stretching* - occurs when a muscle is pulled to a position of increased tension *prior to* the start of a contraction.
9. *Resistance in a Position of Full Muscular Contraction* - resistance must be provided in a position of full contraction to involve the greatest number of muscle fibers in the effort.
10. *Unrestricted Speed of Movement* - the possibility to perform exercise at any speed.

The benefits of full-range exercise speak for themselves:

- A muscle that is optimally strong throughout a complete range of motion can better generate force at any angle requested by the nervous system – which helps performance.

- A muscle with full-range strength can better resist force at all angles – which prevents injury.
- An adequate resistance applied to a muscle in a full-contracted position promotes strength gain.
- An adequate resistance applied to a muscle in a position of full-extension promotes stretching.

The facts are clear, but misunderstood: *"Free weights are better than machines;" "Body-weight training is superior to free-weight training;" "Muscle isolation never occurs during golf. Therefore, integrative exercise is superior."* It's good to have an opinion, but better to have an education. There should be no discussion related to resistance quality, and no excuse when someone places the most productive form of exercise - a quality machine – on the endangered species list, or on the performance-training *delete* list.

In the summer of 1962, offensive guard and ninth-round draft-pick from Lehigh University, Reed Bohovich, received a welcome package from the New York Giants before pre-season training. The starting kit included a plastic bag which housed what appeared to be a skipping rope with instructions. At twenty, the youngest man ever to play in the NFL was expected to report to camp in excellent physical condition by proper use of the enclosed *isometric rope*. Football had yet to discover barbells. Today, conditioning with an isometric rope wouldn't land a job at the peanut stand, but it might yet find its way into sports-performance training.

If a caddy handed you a two-iron in a greenside bunker you would likely hand it back, or send him home. It's not the right tool. Yet, not a word is said when a trainer hands a client an inferior or inappropriate tool on the gym floor. After all, a trainer should know, and a client should trust. If the trainer is relatively new to the field, however, he or she may: *One*, know nothing about *quality of resistance*, other that what's in current use; *Two*, have been led to believe that old-school strength training is not *functional*; or *Three*, may honestly believe that he or she *is* providing the best for the client.

The following chart (Figure 2) compares popular exercise offerings and their ability to deliver what Arthur Jones called *a perfect form of exercise*.

Figure 2: Requirements for Full-Range Exercise

Requirements for Full-Range Exercise	Barbells	BodyWt	TRX	Bands	Pulleys	PowerPlate	Nautilus
Rotary Form Resistance	No	No	No	No	No	No	Yes
Direct Resistance	No	No	No	No	No	No	Yes
Variable Resistance	No	No	No	No	No	No	Yes
Balanced Resistance	No	No	No	No	No	No	Yes
Positive Work	Yes	Yes	Yes	Yes	Yes	Yes	Yes
Negative Work	Yes	Yes	Yes	Yes	Yes	Yes	Yes
Stretching	Yes/No	Yes/No	Yes	Y/N	Yes/No	Yes/No	Yes
Pre-Stretching	Yes	Yes	Yes	Y/N	Yes	Yes	Yes
Resistance in Full Contraction	Yes/No	Yes/No	No	Y/N	Yes/No	Yes/No	Yes
Unfettered Movement Speed	Yes	Yes	Yes	Yes	Yes	Yes	Yes

None of the popular choices of golf performance programs conform, which means that approximately 80 percent of golfers (as indicated on Hole #11) receive partial-range exercise, partial-range fatigue, partial-range results and partial-range protection from injury.

And you thought you were getting your money's worth.

Exercise Form

The proper use of exercise tools is as critical to success as the quality of resistance provided by the tools. Range of motion during exercise can be limited by equipment, but is generally determined by the form or mobility of the trainee. Often, capable trainees do *not* perform exercise through a complete range of motion. Some use a resistance they cannot safely handle in good form, or attempt to perform more repetitions than they realistically can with a challenging weight. Many don't know what to do, or lack proper supervision. When I rarely see a chin-up or push-up performed properly - at a controlled speed or through a full range-of-motion - I wonder what we missed in grade school.

Logically:

- Poor form on lousy equipment fails to produce best results.
- Poor form on good equipment fails to produce best results.
- Good form on lousy equipment fails to produce best results.
- Good form on good equipment produces best results.

Serious golfers insist on the best equipment to suit their game, and on the best tools for the job. The great Nick Weslock, to be certain, polished his fourteen choices. But often, the same group is not as perceptive when selecting the best exercise system or tools to improve the muscles that make it happen. The next time a trainer hands you a latex band to strengthen a golf muscle, tell him or her to get serious. You are.

The next hole introduces a time-tested approach that focuses on strengthening muscles that create the movement, rather than on the movement itself.

References

1. Ellington Darden, *Strength Training Principles* (Winter Park, FL: Anna Publishing, 1977), 74.

Hole #13: 394 Yards, Par 4

REAL FUNCTIONAL TRAINING

I was yards away when the announcer braced for the call, *"Ladies and gentlemen, now on the tee from Kitchener, Ontario, two-time Canadian Amateur Champion, 1966 Canadian PGA Champion, eight-time winner on the Canadian tour ..."* The introduction went on and on, but before the word *gentlemen* pierced the air, Moe Norman had already hit. And before the announcer exhausted his list of accolades, Moe was eighty yards down the fairway, a can of Coke® in one hand and a driver in the other. The driver was face-up - at arm's length - with a ball bouncing off its surface at a pace that matched everything but the stride of its owner. Moe repeated phrases between swigs of Coke and glanced quickly left and right - relaxed now that the ropes had increased his distance from the crowd. He continued his antics until he reached his ball in the middle of the fairway, where it always was. A quick club-exchange with the caddy, a millisecond to plant his feet and *phew*, off he raced to a twenty-foot birdie putt that did not attract a single glance before its execution. Next hole.

The man who shot fifty-nine three times in competition (one with a three-putt; another at the age of sixty-three), and sixty-one four times in a single season, was unique. Not only did he routinely sleep in his car and play golf with ease, his first-hole antics at the St. George's Golf Club in Toronto during the Canadian Open that Sunday in 1968 clearly demonstrated his ability to multitask. Moe could make *complex* look easy. His approach to the game was simple and effective - the way golf training should be.

Simple

The TPI program is anything but. Its insistence on training movement in tandem with muscles that create movement, saddles it with the task of addressing every aspect of a complex skill. Every exercise, drill and stretch is aimed at a specific piece of the puzzle – which sounds thorough, but may be as much a part of the problem, as it is the solution. Input may surface during play.

As a novice, I took weekly group lessons at the club and, during winter months, at an indoor facility on the second floor of an old building in downtown Welland, Ontario. Beyond that, I was on my own. By the time I arrived in Caracas in 1976, I went from not being able to afford a private lesson to not being able to afford golf. Membership fees for a private club (only three in the city, and no public venues) ranged from $250,000 to $450,000 – nothing a school teacher could afford. And so, other than an occasional invitation, I didn't play.

One day, with a little money in my pocket, I called the head professional at the Caracas Country Club for a lesson at his new learning center on the penthouse floor of an executive building in the nearby suburb of Chacaito. Jim Rue was a competent teacher, but I quickly learned I could not handle a lesson. Within five minutes, my head swirled with so many ideas – head, shoulder, left side, takeaway - I couldn't swing. I hadn't learned to play that way.

Too much information during a lesson (or swing) generally leads to disaster. The same applies to golf performance programs. Knowledge of a weak left side, a hitch in your right hip, a surplus of shoulder flexibility on your backswing or a tight rotator cuff can rear its ugly head on the practice tee or course, and add to the burden. Much of the information in the TPI program relates to movement, and movement relates to skill – a component that should be addressed by golf professionals. The physical component should remain in the hands of competent trainers, and both should be kept simple.

Effective

Moe Norman's swing was not attractive, but it worked. As such, it mirrors the training approach proposed in *Golf Performance Training ... What They Won't Tell You*:

1. *Select the muscles used in the swing.*
2. *Strengthen them with the best equipment available, without regard to their intended use.*
3. *Take your new tools (muscles) to the course and apply them to your skill.*

Training to reach your functional potential in any sport, including golf, is not as complicated as some would have you believe, as illustrated by the following:

- In 1972, Bill Bradford was relieved of his duties as football coach at Deland High School in Florida. Impressed by the results Arthur Jones had produced with *negative-only* exercise in *The Quonset Hut*, a makeshift facility behind the school used to train athletes visiting Nautilus Sports/Medical Industries in nearby Lake Helen, Bradford decided to start a weightlifting team. *"At the time,"* claimed Jones, *"I doubt that he really knew the difference between a barbell and a palm tree, but he was not stupid."* The plan was twofold: Build raw strength through the exclusive use of negative exercise (*lowering*, instead of *lifting* weights); and practice the lifting techniques required in competition. The exercise part was simple: *"Two weekly workouts, only one set of each exercise, from six to eight repetitions in each set."* The rest is in the books. With no prior history in the sport, Bradford's team went undefeated and untied for seven consecutive seasons. The non-conventional approach – to strengthen muscles used in the sport, and then practice the sport – was as new to weightlifting as the use of negative-only exercise.

Coach Bradford *was* smart: He quit while he was ahead. His successor started losing because, according to Jones, *"...he went back to using conventional methods. And having been regularly trounced by Bradford's team for seven years, how many other coaches adopted his training method?*

None. Why not? Damned if I know; but I do know that it is impossible to explain insanity."

- In 1975, Arthur Jones sold a set of Nautilus machines to the United States Military Academy (West Point, N.Y.) and agreed to a joint venture, as described by Captain James A. Peterson, Associate Professor of Physical Education: *"The study was designed to provide USMA with the institutional knowledge of how to properly use its Nautilus equipment; to examine the elative effectiveness of different methods of strength training; and finally, (and perhaps, most importantly) to identify the consequences of a short duration, high intensity strength training program."*[1] Peterson designed and directed the study, and claimed, *"...every effort was made to make 'Project Total Conditioning' the most productive and inclusive field research endeavor ever undertaken in the area of strength training."* It was. Jones would have it no other way.

The project involved, among other things, preparation of part of the football team for the upcoming season. At the time, the team practiced twice a day, ran two miles on the track (three times per week, for time) and performed an *unsupervised* circuit of strength-training three times per week. The plan was to train part of the team in a non-traditional fashion – using a *supervised* circuit of strength training on Nautilus machines. Fifty-three cadets were divided into three groups: a Nautilus-Only group (twenty-one); a Control group (sixteen); and a Neck-Only group (sixteen), to verify the effectiveness of prototype neck machines. The Nautilus-Only group, reduced to nineteen by illness and a single football injury, was allocated a two-week trial period to minimize the effect of motor learning. During the trial (and study), the group performed one set of 8-12 repetitions to muscle failure on ten Nautilus machines, three times per week. At the end of the trial period, Captain Peterson and his staff performed the initial testing – strength, flexibility, body composition, etc. Jones contacted Dr. Kenneth Cooper from Dallas, Texas to test and measure cardiovascular outcomes. When Cooper's team of experts arrived, Jones left town. He did not want the results to appear *influenced*.

The procedures for training were *"explicitly objective and precisely controlled,"* but the training itself was brutal – a non-stop circuit of high-intensity exercise that Jones called *Proper Strength Training*. Cadets were pushed to momentary muscle failure at every station, and rushed to the next. *"For all practical purposes,"* claimed Peterson, *"the intensity of the workouts was so severe that it would have been impossible to appreciably extend them. During the first workouts a few of the subjects became nauseated, but after several weeks of training, not only had such negative reactions entirely disappeared, but the average time to complete a comparable workout had been considerably shortened."*[2]

The results of the study astounded those who measured them. After six weeks of training, the Nautilus-Only group increased the resistance used in their exercises (same sequence and number of repetitions as the first workout) by an average of 58.54 percent. At the same time, cadets in the Nautilus-Only group decreased their training time per session by between 4.5-9 minutes, with the average workout lasting just less than thirty minutes.

Coaches and athletes often ignore strength training for fear of losing flexibility. In this study, Proper Strength Training resulted in flexibility gains that were 8-11 *times* that of the Control group on three measures: trunk flexion, trunk extension and shoulder flexion. The average increase with the Nautilus-Only group (on three measures) was 11 percent; the Control group, .85 percent.

Cardiovascular fitness was measured under three conditions: *at rest, during sub-maximal work* and *during maximal work*. On sixty different tests, the Nautilus-Only group was superior to the Control group by a margin that Dr. Kenneth Cooper called *impossible*. At the time, he believed strength training had little or no cardiovascular value - and was dead wrong. According to Captain Peterson's summary: *"The data suggests that some of these cardiovascular benefits apparently cannot be achieved by any other type of training."*

In regard to body composition, the Nautilus-Only cadets lost more body fat than those in the Control group.

The results of Project Total Conditioning, as detailed in the *Athletic Journal* (Vol. 56 September, 1975), were as *functional* as they were spectacular. Apart from the scientific evaluations, the study featured three performance tests: In a two-mile run on the track, the Nautilus-Only group improved more than four (4.32) *times* that of the Control group, lowering their time by eighty-eight seconds, compared to twenty; in a forty-yard dash, the Nautilus-Only group prevailed by improving nearly *twice* (1.89x) that of the Control group; and in a vertical-jump test, the Nautilus-Only group was more than four *times* (4.57x) better than the Control group.

"The study made it clear," concluded Peterson, *"that high-intensity (weight) training is the most efficient conditioning method known that simultaneously develops high degrees of aerobic and anaerobic conditioning. It offers increases in* (muscle) *size and strength, as well as cardiovascular improvement."*[3]

The application of Project Total Conditioning to golf is clear to everyone but functional and TPI trainers. Golf does *not* require you to jump higher or run faster - unless your goal is to match Moe Norman stride for stride - but it has a strength, flexibility, body-composition and, to a lesser degree, cardiovascular component. Adherence to a similar, simple program of exercise can significantly affect performance in golf. Yet, I doubt it will happen.

Despite the success of its outcome, Project Total Conditioning attracted limited interest: It was brutally hard, and bucked tradition. Machine training was *new*, and new to football. The concepts of *high-intensity, muscle failure* and *brief* were new to training. And if you think minor skill change is difficult, try changing the traditions of a sport, or an industry. The coaching community had a better way, just as functional advocates believe they have a better way. They don't.

If a similar study was conducted today (to borrow the phrase of Captain Peterson) *"to examine the elative effectiveness of different methods of strength training; and (more importantly) to identify the consequences of a functional training program,"* it wouldn't be close. The potential for increased strength, flexibility, cardiovascular condition, injury-protection and body-composition results through functional training would be *Pitiful* with a capital *P*, and worse than traditional studies *before* Project Total Conditioning ... with one exception. The skill gained through functional training would equal that gained by Proper Strength Training - *None*.

Hole #14 introduces an exercise program based on the principles of *Proper Strength Training* that will prepare you to play better golf.

References

1. James A. Peterson, "Total Conditioning: A Case Study," *Athletic Journal* 56, no. 9 (1975).
2. James A. Peterson, "Total Conditioning: A Case Study," *Athletic Journal* 56, no. 9 (1975).
3. James A. Peterson, "Total Conditioning: A Case Study," *Athletic Journal* 56, no. 9 (1975).

Hole #14: 429 Yards, Par 4

PROPER STRENGTH TRAINING FOR GOLF

"How to make a rabbit stew; first, you catch a rabbit ..."
Arthur Jones

A kinesiology assignment during my junior year at McMaster University required a detailed analysis of the muscles used in a sport-related movement. Golf was my choice ... and a poor one. By the time I finished, my neck was in my left ear, my butt faced forward and no reader could make contact with anything that resembled a ball. The effort was a dismal failure, but I somehow passed the course - which provided the first of two satisfying moments. The second was the realization that such a project is beyond the scope of the most qualified biomechanical expert. And if I'm wrong, what use would it serve?

Performance-training advocates believe otherwise. The muscles used to pull a golf club down from its apex during a swing, they say, are the same that pull a weight from a high-connection on a pulley station in the gym. And better yet: With proper positioning, the resistance can be pulled along the *same* path as the swing itself to ensure strengthening *exactly* the right muscles in *exactly* the right motion. Arthur Jones best described the fallacy, *"When you're a hammer, everything looks like a nail."*

To simplify the design of a golf-conditioning program, I'll work from two assumptions:

1. The golf swing is a complex movement that *likely* involves every muscle in the body. Therefore, on a broad scale, strengthening *any*

muscle may help the final product (which justifies the reported success of some idiotic routines I've seen over the years).

2. Large muscle groups (*versus* small) make a greater contribution to the success of activities that involve gross-motor movement - such as golf.

Both assumptions simplify the identification of the most important muscles used in the swing:

*   The large muscles of the hip.
*   The large muscles of the lower body: front thigh, rear thigh and calf.
*   The large muscles of the upper body: chest, shoulders and upper back.

And, of less importance:

*   The small muscles of the upper and lower arms: biceps, triceps and forearms.
*   The small muscles of the torso (core): low back, obliques (sides) and abdomen.

The muscles selected must then be connected to strength exercises, as follows:

Figure 1: Prime Movers	Exercise Examples
Hip	
Buttocks (Gluteus)	Hip Extension, Leg Press, Squat
Lower Body	
Front Thigh (Quadriceps)	Leg Extension, Leg Press, Squat
Rear Thigh (Hamstrings)	Leg Curl
Lower Leg (Calf)	Calf Raise
Upper Body	
Chest (Pectorals)	Chest Fly, Chest Press, Dips
Shoulders (Deltoids)	Lateral Raise, Overhead Press
Upper Back (Lats)	Pullover, Lat Pull-Down, Chin-Ups, Rowing

Figure 1: Prime Movers (cont'd)	Exercise Examples
Front Upper-Arm (Biceps)	Pull-Downs, Chin-ups, Rowing, Biceps Curls
Rear Upper-Arm (Triceps)	Chest/Shoulder Press, Dips, Triceps Extensions
Forearm	Wrist Curls, Reverse Wrist Curls
Torso	
Low Back (Erector Spinae)	Lumbar Extension
Sides (Obliques)	Torso Rotation
Front (Abdominals)	Abdomen Curls or Crunches

The exercises must then be linked to the best equipment at your disposal, and sequenced according to established strength training principles. The sample workouts that follow assume the availability of quality exercise machines:

	Workout A (*In Order*)	Workout B	Workout C
1.	Leg Extension	Squat	Hip Extension
2.	Leg Press	Leg Curl	Leg Extension
3.	Leg Curl	Leg Extension	Leg Curl
4.	Calf Raise	Calf Raise	Calf Raise
5.	Lat Pull-Down	Pullover	Lateral Raise
6.	Chest Press	Lat Pull-Down	Overhead Press
7.	Rowing	Chest Fly	Chin-Ups
8.	Lateral Raise	Chest Press	Dips
9.	Triceps Extension	Biceps Curl	Rowing
10.	Biceps Curl	Overhead Press	Abdomen Curl
11.	Lumbar Extension	Torso Rotation	Torso Rotation
12.	Abdomen Curl	Wrist Curl	Reverse Wrist Curl

Sample workouts D, E, and F assume the availability of free-weights and/ or a multi-station pulley:

	Workout D (*In Order*)	**Workout E**	**Workout F**
1.	One-Leg Squat	Squat	Deadlift
2.	Two-Leg Squat	Deadlift	Squat
3.	One-Leg Calf Raise	Sissy Squat	Calf Raise
4.	Two-Leg Calf Raise	One-Leg Calf Raise	Front Raise
5.	Lat Pulldown (Pulley)	Overhead Press	Overhead Press
6.	Chest Press	Chin-Ups	Bent-Arm Pullover
7.	Rowing (Pulley)	Chest Press	Negative Chin-Ups
8.	Lateral Raise	Rowing (Pulley)	Chest Fly
9.	Triceps Extension	Dips	Negative Dips
10.	Biceps Curl	Biceps Curl	Abdomen Curl
11.	Wrist Curl	Torso Rotation (Pulley)	Back Extensions (Roman Chair)
12.	Abdomen Curl	Wrist Curl	Reverse Wrist Curl

Exercise Choice

Properly performed, sample workouts A through F yield excellent results, but exercise selection is flexible. Any upper-back exercise, for example, could be substituted for another. If physical ability limits or prohibits the use of a particular exercise, select an alternative. If injury is involved, seek the advice of a therapist or doctor before attempting an exercise, and modify as needed. The identification of basic movements for each muscle group is an attempt to keep things simple. As you advance, you may wish to substitute, or combine non-listed exercises.

Workouts A, B and C are comprised of approximately 4-6 exercises for the lower body and 6-8 for the upper body, a total of twelve. Despite the importance of the lower body to the golf swing, free-weight routines D, E and F limit the number of exercises for legs and hips: Beyond a few basic movements, there are not many choices. Lunges and step-ups are excluded because it is difficult to hold enough weight in your hands to effectively stimulate lower-body growth. For those who believe otherwise, I quote from Jones' autobiography, "*...while it is neither my intention nor my desire to insult anybody. I am not trying to please anybody either.*" And, for those concerned that one set of twelve exercises is not enough for best results, I remind them of the long list of athletes unable to complete the task in the early 1970's. Properly performed and supervised, it's plenty.

The sample workouts also follow a general pattern: They work large muscles first, then small. It is difficult to summon the energy necessary to stimulate muscles that make the greatest ripple in the pond when your system has been depleted by prior exercise for smaller muscle groups.

The first 8-9 exercises are the meat and potatoes of each workout; the last few, the dessert. Some muscles are a *must-do* each session – buttocks, front thigh, rear thigh, calves, upper back, chest, shoulders and upper arms. Their efforts to exhaustion better shock the body into growth, and can be adequately addressed by one or two direct or indirect exercises per workout. A leg press, for example, is an *indirect* exercise for the buttocks, front thigh and rear thigh. It can be combined with - and preceded by - a *direct* exercise for the same muscles (*in order: hip extension or leg curl or leg extension, and then leg press*). In the same way, shoulder and chest presses present a greater challenge to the triceps muscle of the upper arm than the larger muscles of the shoulder and chest, and can be considered a triceps choice for the day. Workout C (above) has no designated exercise for the muscles of the upper arm, yet two biceps and two triceps challenges lay hidden in the execution of four torso movements.

We have completed four important stages:

1. Identification of the major muscles used in golf.
2. Selection of exercises to strengthen them.
3. Choice of an appropriate tool for the task.
4. And creation of an exercise sequence that best serves our objective(s).

Let's review the guidelines that get us from A to B - the Strength Training Principles introduced on Hole #5 - summarized below:

Figure 2: Strength Training Principles

- Perform one set of twelve exercises: 4-6 for the lower-body and 6-8 for the upper-body.
- Select a resistance that allows 8-12 repetitions.
- Continue each exercise to a point of momentary muscle failure.
- When twelve or more repetitions are performed in perfect form, increase the resistance by 5 percent during the next session.
- Exercise larger muscle groups first, and proceed to smaller.
- Raise the weight to a two count; lower the weight to a four count. When in doubt about speed of movement, move more slowly.
- Attempt to increase repetitions or resistance at every workout; but never sacrifice form in an attempt to achieve 'one more rep.'
- Train no more than three times per week. Allow at least forty-eight hours, but no more than ninety-six hours, between workouts.
- Keep accurate records: Date, resistance, repetitions and total workout time.
- The entire workout should take 20-30 minutes.

Two ingredients produce best results from exercise: good form and high levels of intensity. Further examination of the training principles from the perspectives of form, intensity and progression will lead to a better understanding of their role in the process.

Form

Regardless of equipment, form is often the difference between very good results and no results at all. Since many current trainees believe that exercise performed on the floor provides the greatest opportunity for strength increase, I have yet to see anything approaching proper form.

The lousy performance of simple, schoolyard exercises verifies what Jones espoused in his seminars, *"Ninety-five percent of the people in this country who perform progressive resistance exercise do not know how to lift or lower one repetition of any exercise."*

Everyone talks good form. Few back it up.

Good form starts with proper position:

Stand tall, sit upright or otherwise establish a secure exercise posture before you begin. When using a machine, set the seat at the proper height and fasten the seat belt (if provided) to better target the muscle(s) trained. Make certain the joint system of the working muscle is aligned with the rotational axis of the machine (where possible), and assure that your station is clear of hazards.

Good form ends with a slow speed of movement that keeps tension on the muscle throughout:

A slow speed of movement makes exercise *harder*; and anything that makes exercise harder, makes it more productive. How slow? Use a speed that allows you to *feel the muscle work through every inch of the movement*. Most trainees are surprised by how slow that is. To add an ignored but important point, a *slow* speed during exercise decreases the chance of injury, which is one reason Jones believed it was *impossible* to lift weights too slowly.

Case in point: One day in Caracas, an orthopedic physician mentioned that his training partner, another MD, fell backwards and hit his head on the floor when he caught his heel on something during a standing biceps curl with a barbell. Years later, the two invited me to the scene of the crime, where their volatile form more than warranted use of a hard hat.

Intensity

The intensity of effort must be high to stimulate change:

Arthur Jones viewed the concepts of intensity and duration as follows:

More than a century ago, by a study of the bones of men who spent their lives at manual labor, it was determined that the intensity of work is a factor of great importance; even the chemical composition of the bones is changed by hard work. How much you work – the actual 'amount' of work – is a factor of only secondary importance, and then usually in a negative sense. In effect, 'hard work' is a desirable factor – and a large 'amount of work' is an undesirable factor.[1]

Intensity is a percentage of momentary ability. Maximum intensity occurs when a muscle produces as much pulling force as it momentarily can. With that, the muscle recruits more of its fibers *and* its largest fibers to the effort, increasing the odds of stimulating change.

Intensity can be measured under two circumstances only: during zero effort, and during a full effort. Zero effort is of no value to exercise; 100 percent paves the way to growth stimulation.

At the practical level, maximum intensity manifests itself in two ways: *One*, by reaching *momentary muscle failure* during exercise - the inability to move against resistance despite a full effort; and *Two*, resting less between efforts. The latter engages the cardiovascular system and is less important to golf.

Intensity dictates the duration and frequency of workouts:

Hard work mandates two things: you won't last long, and you will require more recovery time between efforts. Since hard is a *good thing*, productive workouts must be brief, infrequent and provide maximum stimulation with minimal impact (*or inroad*) on the system's recovery ability.

High-intensity exercise decreases the possibility of injury:

When a muscle *fails*, its strength has been diminished to the point that it can no longer produce a force that could exceed its structural limits. Therefore, the final repetitions of an exercise are, by far, *least* likely to cause injury - the opposite of what most trainees believe and feel.

Progression

Try to increase the number of repetitions or the amount of resistance used during each workout, but keep your repetition range at 8-12:

Good results from strength training imply an attempt to progress during every workout. A muscle will *not* grow without stimulation, and stimulation can only occur when a muscle is challenged to exceed its current capacity.

In general, if you cannot perform eight repetitions in good form, the weight is too heavy. If you can perform twelve repetitions or more in good form, the resistance should be increased by approximately 5 percent for the next workout.

Don't finish a set of exercise because you have reached twelve repetitions:

Twelve is an upper guide, *not* a magic number. Where viable, continue until full-range movement is no longer possible. If that number exceeds twelve, adjust the weight accordingly.

Never increase resistance at the expense of form:

Muscles know when an exercise weight has been increased. They sense the difference and respond predictably: *Let's move a little faster to reduce the load.* Within months, form that was once *good* and *slow* deteriorates into something unrecognizable –often without awareness. Have your form reviewed from time to time by a qualified trainer.

Control as many variables as possible:

During MedX certification courses at the University of Florida in the late 1980's, I was confronted each morning by a bold sign at the head of the classroom: *Thou Shalt Standardize.* As with the ultimate result of a golf swing, the quality of a test or exercise outcome depends upon control of as many variables as possible. True progress occurs when repetitions and/ or resistance increases, and other variables remain *fixed.* When factors are not controlled, false impressions appear.

The number of repetitions performed during a workout, for example, may increase because the speed of movement or sequence is different. This is why it is important to select a basic or favorite workout that you perform every month or every two weeks so that valid comparisons can be made. In most gym settings, the only way to determine progress is to compare one performance with another *under the same conditions* of speed, sequence, time of day, resistance, workout duration, etc. An accurate training log helps establish daily, weekly and long-term goals.

Muscle Strength = Muscle Endurance:

A swing with a driver may require the brain to solicit 30 percent of an involved muscle's strength for the effort (leaving 70 percent in reserve for future efforts). When the involved muscle increases in strength, the same swing or effort may require an input of only 20 percent of its capacity (leaving 80 percent in reserve). Increased strength paves the way to increased endurance. Furthermore, research negates the assumptions that performing fewer repetitions with heavy weights is best for strength; and that performing more repetitions with lighter weights is best for local muscle endurance.

With that established, the danger involved in a typical strength test – how much you can lift one time - can be avoided by comparing performances of an equal number of repetitions (from 8-12).

Perform less exercise as strength increases:

Growth slows as you approach your strength potential – generally a sign of lack of stimulation, or inadequate systemic recovery. If the body's reserves are constantly depleted by too much exercise, no growth can occur. The general workout frequency recommended for untrained subjects is three times per week. Following 4-6 months of training, the frequency *must* be reduced. The energy expenditure of workouts at that point creates a greater demand on the body's ability to recover. Less frequency allows more time to compensate. Research reported on Hole #5 supports effective training twice per week.

When Jones encountered plateaus in his own workout regimen, he always reduced the *amount* of exercise, which allowed his system to better recover. He then applied the same principle to the programs of hundreds of bodybuilders and athletes with resounding success.

Other Considerations

Work all the major structures of the body together:

"For best results from exercise", said Jones, *"all of the major muscular structures should be worked – ALL OF THEM, you certainly can build large arms without working your legs – but you will build them much larger, and much quicker, if you also exercise your legs."*[2]

The human body is subject to greater shock when all major muscles are exercised in the same workout. The popular *split* routine is the equivalent of sleeping for your thighs or eating lunch for your calves. When selected parts are exercised, the overall shock is less per workout, which encourages an increase in training frequency to cover all the parts - a step in the wrong direction.

Select exercises that provide the greatest range of motion for the major muscle groups involved in your sport:

In general, the larger the mass of muscle involved in an exercise, the greater the value of the exercise. If there is a choice, select exercises that move the targeted muscle through the greatest range of motion against resistance.

I had the honor of training Jack Nicklaus on several occasions following his hip replacement. We worked around his problem, focused on major muscle groups — front and rear thighs, glutes, calves, chest, shoulders, back and upper arms — and used the finest equipment available at the time, MedX® machines. We also exercised the small muscles of the *core* - obliques and lumbar extensors - on MedX medical tools; and abdominals on a MedX gym machine - as per protocol, infrequently.

The focus on large muscle groups was standard procedure in our golf program, and made sense to those involved. Not today. The majority of trainees (many of them good golfers) and the majority of exercise programs (in gyms, on television, in magazines and books) claim the ability to reach performance potentials by focusing on small muscle groups – the equivalent of performing wrist curls alone to lose excess bodyweight. Not likely.

Perform one set of approximately twelve exercises: 4-6 for the lower-body; 6-8 for the upper body:

From the beginning, Jones sought to discover *"the minimum amount of exercise that produced the maximum result."* For the first twenty years, he performed four sets of each exercise; for the next ten, two sets; and finally, one set to muscle failure. At each step, *less* exercise produced *more* results. Anything more than the minimum was wasted effort at best, and overtraining at worst.

When he launched his commercial endeavor, he invited *anyone in the world* to try his novel approach – a circuit of four *Nautilus Time Machines*, and a handful of Universal-machine and free-weight stations, twelve in all. Jones believed that one or two exercises per muscle group, properly performed, was all that was needed, and all anyone could stand. He was right. The first person to finish the brief circuit - four years later - was Europe's cross-country ski champion. Everyone else ended on the floor, the fortunate ones face-up - some on second and third attempts.

The same occurred in Caracas. Of thirty bodybuilders that entered my facility the first year, one made it to the fifth exercise; the others barely made it to the bathroom.

Recent research (reported on Hole #5) verifies the effectiveness of one set of twelve exercises.

Work large muscles first and small muscles last, in sequence - Hips, legs, torso, arms, abdomen and others:

Training large muscle groups first, while they are fresh, allows the body to recruit a greater number of muscle fibers during work. And work taken to a point of muscle failure creates a greater impact on the system. Ask a bodybuilder who trains in parts which day he most dreads: *Legs* is the answer, because of the impact it has on the system. For proof, train your body in reverse order. You may get more out of the first few exercises, but by the time you reach the lower-body you will have emptied the tank. The net result is a smaller ripple in the pond. And while it's never a bad idea to *change things up*, stimulating large muscles early in the program is more likely to produce best results.

> *Perform brief workouts (20-30 minutes with machines; 30-45 with free weights):*

In the early 1970's, the recommendation of three thirty-minute high-intensity workouts per week was a far cry from the twenty-plus hours commonly performed by bodybuilders. Years later - for better results - Jones modified his stance to twice a week, a thirty-minute total. The brief, infrequent concept, however, was not embraced: Trainees failed to connect *less* exercise to *more* results.

> *Allow a minimum of forty-eight hours and no more than ninety-six hours rest between workouts:*

The body is capable of performing *any* amount of exercise, but not capable of recovering from *any* amount. Both the working muscles *and* the system require time to recover and adapt. While Jones claimed that a muscle exercised to complete failure could recover more than 50 percent of its strength in less than three seconds, he did not infer that total recovery occurs in six seconds. In some cases, recovery may take days or weeks. And while muscle recovery can be rapid, systemic recovery is generally not - and the system feeds the muscle.

When in doubt about frequency, err on the side of *less*.

> *Move as quickly as you can from one exercise to the next as your condition improves:*

A rapid pace between exercises increases the intensity and cardiovascular component of a workout. If you opt to perform aerobic exercise apart from strength training, do your strength training *first* while you are fresh. It has more potential benefits than cardiovascular exercise. An exception may be a trainee whose sport or medical condition prioritizes aerobic activity, not the case with golf.

The limited value of cardiovascular exercise to golf might lead you to believe that moving rapidly *between* strength exercises is not that important. The easy alternative - resting between efforts - can, however, affect the strength component of exercise by reducing the overall shock to the system. Performing twelve exercises in 20 minutes is much more intense than performing the same in twenty-five minutes. Resting between efforts squanders time that could be better spent skill training.

Summary

The Nautilus inventor was open to anything that improved results from exercise. Trial and error led him to believe: *"Everything of any value related to exercise can be stated in less than a thousand words, can, in fact, be fairly well covered in a very few words, as follows: Train hard, train briefly, train infrequently."*[3]

The simplicity of his approach was evident in his second publication, *Nautilus Training Principles: Bulletin #2* (1971), where he outlined a free-weight workout for beginners. From Chapter 34, *"A Simple Example:"*

1. One set of 20 repetitions, full squat
2. One set of 20 repetitions, one-leg calf raises
3. One set of 10 repetitions, standing presses (overhead press)
4. One set of 10 repetitions, regular-grip chins (chin-ups)
5. One set of 10 repetitions, standing presses (a second set)
6. One set of 10 repetitions, regular-grip chins (a second set)
7. One set of 10 repetitions, parallel dips
8. One set of 10 repetitions, standing curls (biceps curls)
9. One set of 10 repetitions, parallel dips (a second set)
10. One set of 10 repetitions, standing curls (a second set)
11. One set of 10 repetitions, stiff-leg deadlifts

The resistance for each exercise was established by trial and error so that the target number of repetitions was barely possible.

Note the similarities between his 1971 suggestions and sample workouts A through F, presented earlier:

- The low amount of exercise compared to the practice of today's trainees.
- The low number of exercises per body part (only seven *different* exercises, above).
- The small number of lower-body exercises (choice is limited with free-weight use only).
- The general sequence of large muscles to small.

The *Simple Example* (above) is more remarkable when you consider that his target audience was bodybuilders, famous for their volume training and *more is better* mind-set. Arthur Jones loved to make people think, but don't be fooled. This beginner's gem - performed to muscle failure with little or no rest between efforts - might force trainees to transfer to the curling program. And it would certainly improve performance in *any* sport, golf included.

In the early 1970's, Nautilus Sports/Medical Industries published suggested routines for athletes in various sports. The following are samples from their golf brochure:

	Basic Workout 1	Basic Workout 2	Basic Workout 3
1.	Hip and Back (Buttocks)	Hip and Back	Hip and Back
2.	Leg Extension	Leg Extension	Leg Extension
3.	Leg Curl	Leg Curl	Leg Press
4.	Pullover	Pullover	Leg Curl
5.	Arm Cross (Chest Fly)	Chin-Ups	Pullover
6.	Lateral Raise (Shoulder)	Arm Cross (Chest Fly)	Arm Cross (Chest Fly)
7.	Rowing Torso (Rowing)	Lateral Raise	Triceps Dips
8.	Biceps Curl	Overhead Press	Rowing Torso (Rowing)
9.	Wrist Curl	Biceps Curl	Biceps Curl
10.	Reverse Wrist Curl	Wrist Curl	Wrist Curl
11.	Abdominal	Reverse Wrist Curl	Reverse Wrist Curl

Observations

More than a decade ago, I wrote that strength training would not come into vogue on the PGA Tour until someone who resembled Mr. Universe won the US Open. As ridiculous as it seemed, the purpose was to *connect* the relationship between muscle strength and golf performance. At the time, Tiger Woods was the referenced Mr. Universe.

I also wrote that doubling the strength of a superior athlete has a greater effect on performance than doubling the strength of the average weekend warrior. The superior athlete has the skills (established nervous system channels) and abilities to better convert the increased strength to a positive outcome.

When Woods set the modern standard of physical preparation, there was a general reluctance to lift weights with any kind of intensity. His dominance forced peers to at least tip-toe into the arena of fitness with cardiovascular activities, stretching and a *bit* of strength training. With a lot at stake, the majority failed to fully commit.

The recent introduction of the TPI program, with its roots in functional training, saved more than a few hind ends – at least on the surface. It was *like* strength training, without slugging weights. It was *like* work, but fun. And it was *like* golf. Through slick marketing, the insult to physiology became the rage, and took reluctant professionals off the hook. A fortunate few did not take the bait.

The August 2014 PGA Championship at Valhalla Golf Club in Louisville, Kentucky resulted in a Rory McIlroy victory that lead TV broadcasters to crown him the next Tiger Woods, using statistics to support their claim. When Rory won the tournament, his third in a row that season, he looked much like Woods - a full chest, muscular arms, and as fit as could be. One announcer stated that he had added six or seven pounds of muscle in the past several months, a possibility. To me, it was a repeat of someone with muscles dominating the field.

The week before, I watched McIlroy *average* 345 yards off the tee down the middle of narrow fairways. One announcer called it *"the finest exhibition of driving I have ever seen."* After one such effort, they showed a side-by-side comparison of his swing to that of a competitor for the purpose of identifying differences in technique. The analysis focused on the transition from backswing to downswing, and highlighted minor discrepancies. The greatest visible difference (not mentioned, and rightly so) was what exited the left sleeve of their golf shirts. Rory had meat; his competitor, yet to be determined. The contrast demonstrated more than met the eye.

Genetics plays a large role in physical potential. In this case - and to be fair - the golfer with the stick-like arms has an *ectomorphic* body frame - less likely to become muscular with *any* kind of training. Woods and McIlroy have *mesomorphic* frames that more easily build muscle. Another point: The player with the small arms exercises in a local facility that endorses functional golf training, using *pro-style fitness tools* - rubber bands and Swiss balls. It is obvious that Tiger and Rory use superior equipment. Neither would acquire their arm size and strength by playing with toys that pretend to be tools. Both realized they would never reach their potential without hard, progressive resistance exercise. TPI workouts may demand a cardiovascular or skill input (*different* skills at that), but they fail to challenge the strength system – the only productive factor in performance. Will golfers - or trainers - ever see the light?

Don't be too hopeful.

Months ago, during the 2015 Honda Classic, a PGA Tour player trained in our facility. It didn't take long to discover his orientation. He sauntered through the gym with a Swiss ball in one hand and resistance bands in the other - wondering why victories were few and far between.

It reminded me of an impression left by a man in a one-piece jump suit on television when I was six years old. The largest man I had ever seen had more energy than a kangaroo. Every day that I hovered over my battlefield of metal soldiers, Jack LaLanne commanded his own legion, *"OK, ladies, one, two, three, four … and one, two, three, four."* I knew nothing about him or what he was doing, but clearly recall: *Why was a big, strong man doing such stupid little things? Surely, he must slip outside and uproot trees during commercial breaks to vent frustration.*

The point is this: Regardless of potential, if you do everything right in a golf program that has roots in functional training, you will become frustrated by a lack of results and initiate, or return to, what you should have been doing all along – proper strength training. Time and again, trainees abandon progressive resistance exercise for a modality with greater appeal, and end up returning because they have lost strength, or failed to gain it at a rate promised by the new activity.

Proper Strength Training establishes a *concrete* base for all sports. Its popularity and acceptance surged in the 1970's and 80's with the introduction of Nautilus machines and the writings of Arthur Jones, but it has since taken a back seat to functional exercise. The ideas that once led trainees to their athletic potential are now *outdated*, *non-functional*, *useless* and even *crazy*.

They are not.

The application of proper strength training to golf, as presented, has been tried and proven – and the desire to produce better results dictates its return. *Crazy?* Ponder this from a friend of Arthur Jones: *"The fact that I am crazy does not prove that you are sane."* (John Peters)

Let's examine several advanced methods of strength training for golf.

References

1. Arthur Jones, *Nautilus Training Principles, Bulletin No. 2* (Self published, 1971), 71.
2. Arthur Jones, *Nautilus Training Principles, Bulletin No. 2* (Self published, 1971), 85.
3. Arthur Jones, "My First Half-Century in the Iron Game," *arthurjonesexercise,* http://www.arthurjonesexercise.com./ First_Half/64.PDF

Hole #15: 336 Yards, Par 4

ADVANCED TRAINING FOR GOLF

Advanced strength training for golf involves the following:

- The use of techniques that increase the odds of stimulating change.
- Difficult sequences that produce a deeper inroad into a muscle's reserve capacity.
- Less exercise.

Training Techniques

Negative Work

According to Arthur Jones, *"Muscles are forty percent stronger lowering than lifting weight."* In effect, if you can lift one hundred pounds in good form, you can lower 140 pounds in a slow, controlled manner. The discrepancy is due to numerous factors: the effect of gravity, friction that exists within exercise machines (when machines are used), and something rarely considered … internal muscle friction. When you lift a weight, the muscle must overcome the weight of the resistance, the pull of gravity, friction inherent in the exercise tool, and friction generated by the movement of muscle-fibers. All factors hinder the lifting phase (you must overcome their resistive force), but assist the lowering phase (by acting as a brake). As a result, the resistance *feels* heavier on the way up, and lighter on the way down. Despite how it *feels*, however, Arthur Jones declared the lowering phase of each repetition more important than the lifting phase – with good reason.

When a muscle is exercised to a point of momentary failure (when it can no longer *lift* a weight through a complete range of motion with a full effort), the depth of fatigue assumes a particular value – *X* amount of inroad. When a muscle is exercised to a point of momentary failure as it *lowers* a weight (lowers in less than three seconds with loss of control), the depth of fatigue (inroad) assumes a greater value – *X* plus 40 percent.

Jones used an analogy to illustrate the practical difference: *"Take an untrained man to the base of a tall building. Have him walk up the stairs to the fiftieth floor and take the elevator down. He will likely experience muscle soreness in the morning. If the same man, under the same conditions, takes the elevator up to the fiftieth floor and walks down, he will be unable to get out of bed in the morning."* Negative work, despite how *easy* it feels by comparison, creates more muscle soreness than normal positive/negative work, attesting to the depth of stimulation encountered – the inroad.

Another point: When you can no longer lift a weight during exercise, you can continue the effort by lowering the weight. Jones developed three practical methods to best apply this information.

In order of difficulty …

Negative-Only Exercise

Negative-only exercise means just that: The positive or lifting phase of the movement is performed by *other* muscles or by external assistance, leaving trainees to perform *only* the negative or lowering phase: Other muscles lift; you lower. The use of external assistance normally requires manpower, unless you are creative. In the 1950's, according to Jones, Tennessee strongman Bob Peoples *"used a negative-only style of exercise; he rigged up a tractor to lift a very heavy weight that he could not lift, and then trained in a negative-only fashion by lowering this heavy weight back down to the bottom position."* While the image is not likely to trigger a stampede of golfers to the maintenance shed, it motivated the Nautilus inventor to investigate the effect of lowering weight on muscle growth. The ultimate spark was provided by his competitors.

In the early 1970's, several equipment manufacturers heralded the benefits of positive-only exercise in a form of technology called *isokinetics* - lifting a resistance at a constant speed controlled by a motorized machine.

The lowering phase of exercise, they claimed, was useless and somehow dangerous. Arthur smelled a rat, and decided to investigate.

In January of 1973, Nautilus employee, Casey Viator, was involved in an industrial accident in which he nearly lost the little finger of his right hand, and almost died from an allergic reaction to a tetanus shot. Jones had successfully trained Viator for the 1971 Mr. America competition and was well aware of his outstanding potential for muscle mass. The twenty-one year old had lost thirty-three pounds of bodyweight as a result of the accident, and was visibly distraught. Jones flew a set of Nautilus machines to Fort Collins, Colorado and arranged a strength-training *experiment*[1] conducted by Dr. Elliot Plese, Ph.D., Director of the Department of Exercise Physiology at Colorado State University. Casey performed one set each of twelve exercises to failure, every other day for twenty-eight days, and produced the following results: a bodyweight gain of 45.28 pounds (from 166.87 to 212.15); a body-fat loss of 17.93 pounds; a body-fat percentage drop from 13.8 to 2.47; and a net muscle gain of 63.21 pounds in fourteen workouts. Although it was clear that Viator was *"rebuilding previously existing levels of muscular size,"* the experiment represented an outstanding example of what can be accomplished with freakish genes and proper training. The training itself proved as unique as the result.

The protocol of what came to be known as *The Colorado Experiment* included three ingredients most trainees, at the time, chose to ignore:

1. Exercise was performed on machines only – no free weights.
2. Exercise was performed in a *Negative-Only* fashion. Viator *never* lifted a weight; he *only* lowered weight.
3. Resistance was lowered to a ten-count.

The results were accurate, verified, supported by film and accomplished in twenty-eight days, which prompted a question I ask self-proclaimed bodybuilders who find the tale hard to believe, *"Did Arnold ever gain 63.21 pounds of muscle in his lifetime?"*

Jones continued his investigation by constructing tools that accurately measured the rate of muscle fatigue during the lifting and lowering phases of exercise - suspecting that the difference in output between the two was due to *internal muscle friction*. He needed proof. His initial studies revealed that, on average, a muscle loses strength at a rate of approximately 2 percent per repetition. That is, ten repetitions of exercise results in a strength loss of approximately 20 percent. He also discovered that positive (lifting) and negative (lowering) strength diminished at similar rates during the first repetitions of exercise, but suspected that the rate accelerated when exercise was taken beyond – when positive strength was reduced by 100 percent. (*Under normal conditions, the body will not allow a muscle to lose 100 percent of its strength for safety reasons: Momentary muscle failure at ten repetitions represents, for most, a strength loss of only 20 percent*). The effort, Jones recognized, would take an extraordinary subject, more repetitions of exercise, an entourage of cheerleaders, weeks of recovery and possibly an ambulance.

His seventeen-year search culminated with an experiment using a highly-motivated, reliable subject, and revealed the following:

- Positive and negative strength diminished at approximately the same rate for 12-13 repetitions.
- When the subject could no longer lift the weight on his own, despite a full effort, the initial drop in negative strength (lowering ability) began to rise. The rise represented an increase of internal muscle friction, which helps you lower.
- *"Reaching that level of fatigue while performing only positive exercise,"* claimed Jones, *"is all but impossible, would require a very high number of sets of the exercise, far too many sets; but reaching that level of fatigue from negative-only exercise is relatively easy."*[2]
- In effect, when positive strength is reduced by 100 percent (a gargantuan effort), the resulting fatigue is equal to that encountered when negative strength is reduced by only 18 percent. This explains why the use of negative-only work is so practical and effective. A little goes a long way.

When Jones first revealed the potential of negative work to the bodybuilding community, many professionals began performing *every* set of *every* exercise at *every* workout in a negative style, and then claimed *it didn't work*, which led Arthur to comment, *"If race horses were trained as much as most bodybuilders train, you could safely bet your money on an out-of-condition turtle – it would be unlikely that a horse trained in such a fashion could even make it around the track, and certainly not rapidly."*

With that in mind, guidelines for negative-only training have been established:

- Select a weight that is 40 percent heavier than normal.
- Have a sufficient number of assistants lift the weight to a full-contracted position. This requires planning and adherence to safety concerns.
- Pass the weight to the trainee in a smooth manner.
- Slowly lower the weight in 10-15 seconds.
- Repeat. Assistants lift the weight, you lower.
  - o *When you can reverse the movement, don't try to.*
  - o *When you can hold the weight motionless, don't try to.*
  - o *When it becomes impossible to stop the movement, try to stop it.*
  - o *Continue until the time of descent occurs in less than three seconds.*
- Perform one set of 6-10 repetitions.

Negative-only is the hardest and most productive form of exercise. It requires a resistance heavier than normal, and a cast of able assistants – they lift, you lower. In the 1970's, bodybuilders and football players, under Jones' guidance, successfully performed negative-only exercise in a makeshift building behind the DeLand (Fl) High School. Eventually, several exercises had to be abandoned due to the risk of transferring heavy weights safely to the trainee.

To resolve the problem of requiring an entourage of assistants, Jones built machines that used the strongest muscles of the body (hips and legs) to lift a heavy weight that was then lowered by smaller upper-body muscles (chest, shoulders and arms). He marketed only a few of the tools due to friction and impracticality - but one became a best seller. The Nautilus Multi-Exercise machine offered, among other exercises, the possibility of performing negative-only chin-ups and dips *without* a training partner.

Three stair-steps in front of an adjustable chin/dip bar allowed trainees to ascend to a contracted position using their legs, and then lower with arms only. It looked easy, but was not. An optional waist-belt clipped to the weight-stack assured that ten negative chin-ups to failure was the equivalent of completing a 100-meter Olympic final – and never wanting to run again.

In the absence of a Nautilus Multi-Exercise machine, negative-only chin-ups and dips can be performed by positioning a bench or set of aerobic steps beneath a chin or dip station. Step to the top position, remove your legs, lower slowly in ten seconds and quickly return to the top using your legs. Avoid jumping to the start position, especially as fatigue sets in. Continue until lowering occurs in less than three seconds, or when you cannot safely control the descent. A spotter is recommended.

Chin/dip assist stations typically found in gyms are not appropriate for negative-only work. The platform is generally too low to safely reach an appropriate starting position.

Negative-Accentuated Exercise

Negative-accentuated exercise requires no supervision and - for that reason alone - may be your best choice of advanced alternatives. It requires the use of exercise machines with a movement arm that allows simultaneous use of both left and right limbs.

Training guidelines follow:

- Select a weight that represents 60-70 percent of your current resistance.
- Lift the weight with both limbs at a normal, slow pace (2-3 seconds). Lower the weight *with one limb only* in 10-15 seconds.
- Lift again with both limbs and lower slowly with the opposite limb.
- Follow the same general guidelines for negative-only exercise: Discontinue when you can no longer lift the weight, control the descent, or when unnatural postures surface.
- Perform one set of 8-12 repetitions (twelve lifts and six lowering movements with each limb).

The Positives: This style of training requires no assistance and allows measurable progress. When the weight transfers to one limb, it represents 120 percent of what you would normally lower.

The Negatives: While one limb works, the other rests and recovers. That, combined with an accumulation of internal muscle friction, may lead to the frustration of slow failure. The transfer of resistance from two limbs to one must be smooth to avoid postural shifts, especially as fatigue sets in.

Negative-Emphasis Exercise

Negative-emphasis involves lifting a weight in a normal fashion and having a training partner apply manual resistance to the movement arm or weight as it lowers. Resisting the added push during the lowering phase increases the inroad and intensity of work per set. The task requires external assistance which introduces variables and a search for someone who can provide a smooth, reliable push. From the assistant's perspective, judgment of how hard to push is determined by *feel* and the speed of the movement arm. In either case, the force applied cannot be accurately measured which makes long-term progress impossible. To add, the application of manual resistance harbors its own problems. Hesitation by trainer or trainee could result in sudden acceleration or deceleration of the working muscle – the definition of injury. Manual resistance must be *softened* when a muscle reaches a stretched position.

Apply the following guidelines:

- Select a machine with a fused movement arm (one that requires use of both limbs together).
- Reduce the standard weight you use by 30 percent.
- Lift normally (in 2-3 seconds), lower slowly (in 10-15 seconds) as you resist the push of a training partner. Repeat.
- Continue until the act of lowering cannot be controlled.
- Perform one set of 6-10 repetitions.

The Positives: The increased emphasis on lowering creates a greater inroad when failure is reached.

The Negatives: The need for a spotter or training partner, the inherent danger of manual pressure and the inability to measure progress limit the use of this technique to it best application – to surpass plateaus on specific exercises.

Summary

Of the three forms of negative work – Negative-Only (NO), Negative-Accentuated (NA) and Negative-Emphasis (NE) – Negative-Accentuated is the only practical choice: It requires no external assistance. Negative-Only is the most effective but has limited application in gyms, and may prove dangerous to spotters. Advanced workouts that involve some form of negative training for every exercise should be restricted to a total of 6-8 exercises. Otherwise, perform a regular workout with select exercises executed in a negative style, as suggested in an early Nautilus golf brochure:

Mixed Workout No. 1	Mixed Workout No. 2
1. Hip and Back	1. Pullover
2. Leg Extension	2. Chin-Ups (NO)
3. Leg Press (NE)	3. Arm Cross or Chest Fly (NE)
4. Hip Adduction	4. Chest Press (NE)
5. Hip Abduction	5. Lateral Raise (Shoulders)
6. Pullover	6. Rowing Torso (Rowing)
7. Chin-Ups (NO)	7. Wrist Curl
8. Arm Cross or Chest Fly	8. Leg Extension (NA)
9. Triceps Dips	9. Leg Curl (NE)
10. Biceps Curl (NE)	10. Calf Lowers
11. Wrist Curl	11. Rotary Torso
12. Rotary Torso	

Negative work is challenging, difficult to recover from, and must be used infrequently. Regardless of style, one set of negative exercise per body part per week is the general recommendation.

More is *not* better.

Positive Work

1¼-Repetitions

Muscle stimulation and strength gain is related to the number of muscle fibers involved in an exercise, and determined by two factors: Intensity of effort and position of the muscle during exercise (*the only position that involves maximum recruitment of muscle fibers is full contraction*). The combination of high intensity and a full-contracted position can be achieved by the performance of 1¼-repetitions on exercise machines that provide adequate resistance in a contracted position.

The Leg Extension machine is a good example.

- Set the machine's resistance to your normal weight or slightly below.
- Lift the weight to the top position and *pause* momentarily.
- Slowly lower the weight about one quarter of the way down. From there, reverse direction and slowly lift the weight again to the top position. *Pause* again.
- Lower the weight to the original starting position.
- One full lift, followed by a one-quarter lift. Repeat until movement is no longer possible.

Use of this technique reduces the number of repetitions normally achieved. Its effectiveness lies in the fact that, on the road to fatigue, the muscle spends more time in - or near - a position of full contraction, which triggers the recruitment of more muscle fibers during the effort.

Its application is limited to exercises that provide resistance in a contracted position. With few exceptions (calf raises, shoulder shrugs, upright row and wrist curls), free-weight exercises do not qualify. Machine exercises that push away from the body's center (squats, presses and dips) are also poor candidates. A *pause* in a contracted position during such movements represents a rest.

Perform a workout that includes as many 1¼-repetition exercises as possible (in a ten-exercise routine) or work the technique into a normal session. Keep accurate records.

Super Slow

The Super-Slow® system of training was developed by former Nautilus employee, Ken Hutchins, who timed the speed of each repetition to improve exercise form by eliminating momentum. His solution: ten seconds to lift, ten seconds to lower; a range of 4-6 repetitions; and brief, infrequent training.

The Positives: A slower pace of movement during exercise ...

- Makes resistance *feel* heavier, which sends a signal to recruit larger muscle fibers.
- Forces a muscle to *work* through its entire range of motion *without* momentum.
- Promotes hard, brief and infrequent training – a step in the right direction.
- Generally produces greater results.

The Negatives:

- Some trainees don't like the rigidity of the system, or the sterile environment of Super-Slow facilities.
- Others reject the large clock *in your face* at each station to keep an accurate account of time.

Super-Slow training is best performed with machines, but not *any* machine will do. Friction reduces the value of slow movement - makes the lifting phase feel heavier and lowering phase feel lighter, which may reduce tension on a working muscle during the latter. The average gym machine has too much internal friction, which prompted Super-Slow facilities to modify low-friction machines to satisfy their needs. In general, gym machines suffice if they are relatively new.

A super-slow cadence can be applied to an entire workout or to select exercises within a workout. If it is implemented in a full-body session, perform no more than eight exercises and limit frequency to once a week. If Super-Slow exercises are used at random, perform no more than four movements in a single workout, and train no more than twice per week.

It doesn't sound like much, but Super-Slow will get your attention. It's a difficult way to train.

Exercise Sequence

Pre-Exhaustion

Simple adjustments to the sequence of exercises can make a significant difference in workout intensity. The goal of pre-exhaustion routines is to force a fatigued muscle to *immediately* perform a second exercise with *fresh* help. A back-to-back leg extension/leg press, for example, forces tired thigh muscles (from the extension) to greater fatigue with help from fresh hip muscles (involved in the press).

Best results with pre-exhaustion combinations occur when time between the two exercises is restricted to less than three seconds because of the rapid initial recovery of a fatigued muscle. Nautilus Sports/Medical Industries constructed several *double* machines in the early 1970's that allowed two exercises from one seat to facilitate the effectiveness of pre-exhaustion training: The Nautilus® Compound Leg (leg extension/leg press), Double Shoulder (lateral raise/shoulder press), Double Chest (chest fly/chest press), Pullover/Torso Arm (pullover/pull-down) and Behind Neck/Torso Arm (behind-neck pullover/behind-neck pull-down). Proper execution on double machines took such a physical toll that recommended use was restricted to no more than two combinations per workout. Unfortunately, double machines are no longer manufactured (more money passes hands by selling single-station machines) which limits pre-exhaustion exercise to moving quickly from one station to another in less than three seconds - a difficult task.

Pre-exhaustion combinations include:

- *Legs* – Leg Extension *immediately* followed by Leg Press or Squat (barbell).
- *Shoulders* – Lateral Raise *immediately* followed by Shoulder (Overhead) Press.
- *Upper Back* – Pullover (free weight or machine) *immediately* followed by Pull-down to front or Chin-ups (both, palms up).

- *Chest* – Chest Fly *immediately* followed by Chest Press (free-weight or machine).
- *Biceps* – Biceps Curls *immediately* followed by Pull-down or Negative Chin-ups (palms up).
- *Triceps* – Triceps Extensions *immediately* followed by Negative Dips or Chest Press.

Guidelines: No more than two pre-exhaustion combinations should be included in a workout of ten total exercises, no more than twice per week.

Non-stop *triple combinations* add a twist to pre-exhaustion training, as follows:

- *Legs* – Leg Press/ Leg Extension/ Full Squat (a favorite of Arthur Jones).
- *Shoulders* – Lateral Raise/ Upright Row/ Shoulder Press.
- *Upper Back* – Pull-down/ Pullover (machine)/ Bent-over or Seated Row. Pull-down/ Pullover (machine)/ Negative Chin-ups.
- *Chest* – Chest Press/ Chest Fly/ Negative Dips.
- *Biceps* – Chin-ups/ Biceps Curls (barbell)/ Negative Chin-ups.
- *Triceps* – Chest Press/ Triceps Extensions/ Negative Dips.

The second and third exercises of each triple combination require a reduction of as much as 40-50 percent of the resistance normally used. Time factors and instructions for its effective use remain the same: No more than two triple combinations in a workout of ten exercises - twice a week at most.

Push/Pull

Another effective sequence, *Push/Pull*, alternates between pushing and pulling movements - a push *away* from your body followed by a pull *towards* it. The sample below is the Nautilus Push/Pull routine I used with Venezuelan bodybuilders on their inaugural exposure to the system (*in order*):

1. Leg Press
2. Leg Extension

7. Chest Press
8. Rowing

3. Leg Curl
4. Hip & Back (glute machine)
5. Shoulder Press
6. Pull-Down (to front, palms up)

9. Negative Dips
10. Negative Chin-Ups
11. Triceps Extensions
12. Biceps Curls

It resembled a non-stop mule kick.

Amount of Exercise

Advanced Training

Without defining 'advanced,' a reduction in training frequency is warranted when workouts begin to deplete recovery ability and halt progress. A brief scan of workout records that compares identical sessions reveals such plateaus. Novice trainees normally take a few weeks to acquire good form, a few months to reach intensity levels that stimulate growth, and several more to reach a plateau. Four to six months of hard, progressive exercise may warrant a reduction in training.

There are two ways to deal with plateaus: Make exercise harder and/or allow the body more time to recover. The majority of this chapter has been dedicated to the former – training methods that make exercise harder. A more extensive list is available in Ellington Darden's 2004 book, *The New High Intensity Training*[3], where he elaborates upon the following:

- *Cheating Repetitions*
- *Forced Repetitions*
- *Breakdown Sets*
- *1¼-Repetitions*
- *Stage Repetitions*
- *Pre Exhaustion Sets*
- *Negative Repetitions*
- *Super-Slow Repetitions*
- *Extremely Slow Repetitions*

Dr. Darden's suggestions are effective, and most do *not* require a training partner.

A reduction in the amount of strenuous physical exercise with advanced trainees extends beyond the realm of strength training. The black-and-white television in the living room of our wartime house on Navy Street in Welland, Ontario allowed me to witness another event that influenced my life. This time, my battlefield and The Jack LaLanne Show surrendered to a familiar name. At the age of six, I watched Roger Bannister break the four-minute mile, but details escape my recall. Apparently, the announcer had a flair for the dramatic, *"As a result of Event Four, the One Mile, was the winner R.G. Bannister of Exeter and Merton Colleges, in a time which, subject to ratification, is a track record, an English Native record, a United Kingdom record, a European record, in a time of three minutes ..."* The eruption drowned what remained. A milestone had been toppled.

At the time, I didn't know who he was or the significance of the event, but he had the same name. That was enough. Months later, I watched Bannister commit the renowned technical error of peering over his inside shoulder to detect the whereabouts of Australian, John Landy, breathing down his neck on the final turn. Bannister looked left; Landy passed to the right – and produced a cloud over my brigade.

The prelude to that earth-shattering event in 1954 was - like all challenges - filled with hard work, planning and heartbreak. The world record had been *on hold* for eight years due to World War II and was held by Swedish runner, Gunder Haegg, in part because Sweden was not involved in the war. Three others - Bannister, Landy and American, Wes Santee - had run 4:02 that year. The closer they came to breaking the four-minute mile, the tougher it became.

Reaching your strength potential presents a similar challenge. Like climbing a mountain, there are many plateaus; and the closer you get, the more difficult it becomes. Bannister was criticized by the press for not training enough (he didn't run during the five days preceding the record attempt). He was busy balancing a medical career with an international track-and-field career and received his medical degree from Oxford six weeks *after* the event. But he knew his body. *"In those days, I didn't train very much,"* he said. *"We didn't really know how to train in modern terms. There was this thing called 'burning yourself out.' I didn't want to burn myself out at eighteen, and I had a notion that if I looked after myself, trained carefully, I would go on improving, not by training two to three hours per day, but by training three quarters of an hour a day. It seemed to me logical that you could go on improving, and you didn't have to spend all day running."*[4]

Without direct reference or knowledge, Roger Bannister understood the basics of advanced strength training. Slow muscle growth reflects either lack of stimulation or - in his words – "...*burning yourself out.*" Following 4-6 months of training (or when plateaus are reached), workout frequency *must* be reduced to accommodate the body's need to recover from the increased demand.

Figure 1 (below) is a theoretical chart demonstrating the progression from initial workout to strength potential. Note the required *decrease* in the amount of exercise performed at each stage.

Figure 1: Reaching Strength Potential

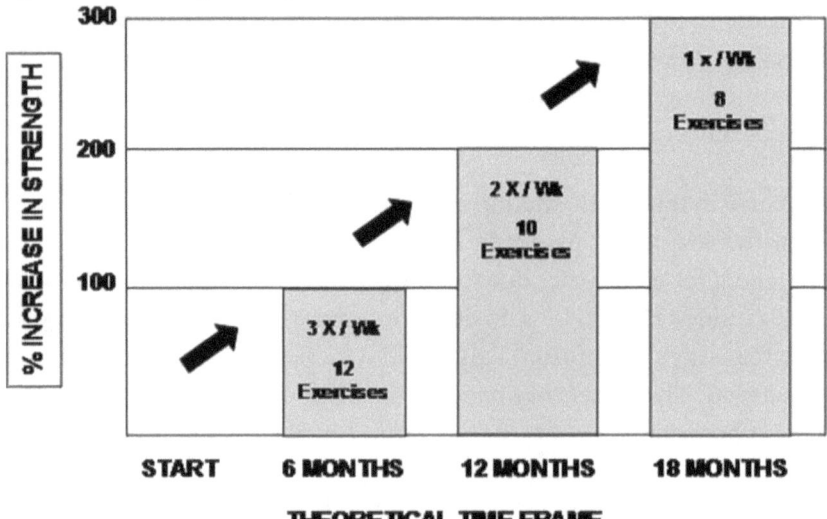

Following a lifetime of progressive resistance exercise, the Nautilus inventor believed that his results would have improved if he had reduced workouts to one brief session per week.

Summary

Advanced training requires less, but harder exercise. Seeking that balance is a trial-and-error process that requires a third ingredient, patience. Growth (as depicted in Figure 1, above) is rarely linear, as described by Arthur Jones:

The human muscular structure is capable of growing at an almost alarming rate, as has been clearly demonstrated in thousands of cases with beginning trainees. It was recently noted in the scientific community that growth occurs in very sudden spurts. A child may increase their height by as much as an inch overnight, literally in a few hours. I noticed the same thing in regard to gains in muscular size over 30 years ago: I have had my arms increase in size by a full inch from the time I went to bed at night until I got up the next morning, and while my increases in size have not always been that great, they have always been sudden, a matter of a few hours at most, and perhaps a matter of a few minutes. I was never able to determine just how much time was actually required for such spurts.[5]

Perhaps Sir Roger encountered one of those spurts on that famous day in 1954.

References

1. Ellington Darden, *The Nautilus Bodybuilding Book* (Chicago, IL: Contemporary Books, 1986), 83.
2. Arthur Jones, "My First Half Century in the Iron Game," Ironman, May (1995), 184.
3. Ellington Darden, *The New High Intensity Training* (New York, NY: Holtzbrinck Publishers, 2004), 137.
4. Academy of Achievement, "Sir Roger Bannister Interview – Academy of Achievement," *achievement.org.*, http://www.achievement.org/autodoc/page/ban0int-7.
5. Arthur Jones, "My First Half Century in the Iron Game," Ironman, December (1993), 176.

Hole #16: 340 Yards, Par 4

AVOIDING HAZARDS

s evolution dictates, the kid from the caddy shack eventually plays golf with the men for whom he carried. It was my turn to step to the plate.

I was paired that Saturday with a man who had taken a similar path – a man who shouldered the bag of Walter Hagan on that same tee during the General Brock Open in 1935.

The eleven-time major champion was in good hands.

The hands belonged to a kid who would go on to win the club championship, work a lifetime in a steel mill, and crush opponents *before* they teed up and *after* they finished.

Steve Kozak looked the part. Rugged and chiseled, he greeted you with a deep voice, vice-like grip and pleasant smile – all of which earned him the name, *Muscles McGurn*.

When we first met, Steve was barely fifty and, in golfing terms, past his prime - but he could play, and I could learn. That day, on the eighth tee - a 180-yard gem that required an uphill shot to a small target - three of us pulled drivers from the bag, believing it wasn't enough. The wind howled like never before. Steve fashioned a two-iron and, in that deep voice, quickly dismissed all slurs from the peanut gallery, *"I'll never hit a G ... D ... wood on a par three."* In turn, he hammered his ball about forty yards short of the green, and mumbled his way up the fairway.

I learned more about Mr. Kozak when the club converted a swampy area to the right of the seventeenth fairway into a pond that was now *in play*. Like a light switch, Muscles McGurn was often seen approaching the seventeenth green from the middle of the adjacent twelfth fairway, far to the left. He would *not* visit that pond. Two years later, the club installed a retainer pond between the twelfth and seventeenth fairways, precisely where he aimed. Leather peered between the fingers of his grip.

Word was out: If there was trouble left, Steve aimed right - way right. If there was trouble on both sides, he chose the lesser of two evils. Muscles McGurn opted for the safe route.

He was not alone.

Due to clever hype, the *safe* approach is prevalent among those who select a program of physical preparation for golf. Lifting weights, many fear, will somehow ruin all they have worked for – derail their success.

Plain and simple, *it will not*; but I'm not the one to decide.

The result is a search for alternatives, a search the field of exercise has both accommodated and confused: *Good* does not ensure longevity, or *lousy* signal demise.

Thus, many of today's offerings are adaptable to the perceived needs of the Royal and Ancient game: Yoga, Pilates, vibration training, suspension training (TRX) and then some. When someone decides how to better use a broomstick, we will likely have *Broomstick for Golf.*

Let's examine the effect of a handful of current offerings on the potential benefits of exercise: Strength, flexibility, cardiovascular condition, body composition and injury prevention. None of the offerings - including proper strength training - have a direct or positive influence on skill.

Suspension Training (TRX)

If the value of exercise is judged by the quality of resistance and the range of motion over which the resistance is effective, TRX training merits an F. Like free-weights, it attempts to apply straight-line force to rotational movement.

The only thing that counts in non-machine exercise is the vertical movement of resistance against the pull of gravity. Any direction but vertical lessens the effect of gravity, and the effectiveness of the exercise. With few exceptions, the black and yellow TRX straps that hang from gym ceilings provide resistance in an arc that rarely travels vertically. As a result, the effective strength curve (the application of resistance to the working muscles) is never correct, and often, the reverse of what it should be. For example, the starting position of the TRX chest press (with arms extended and chest muscles contracted) features body-weight resistance at its minimum. Lowering the chest to a stretch position near the floor increases the resistance to its highest level - where shoulders are most vulnerable to injury; and working muscles, weakest. The effective resistance is the opposite of what it should be. When a muscle is fully contracted the resistance should be at its peak, or at least adequate, to stimulate change.

The same applies to TRX pulling motions. During a standing row (regardless of foot position), resistance is greatest when muscles are stretched and weakest when they are contracted – the opposite of ideal. Close your eyes during *any* TRX exercise, and focus on how it *feels*: Muscles are challenged when they are stretched, and not when they are contracted. From that, you might conclude that TRX training is more likely to produce gains in flexibility than strength, if you can avoid injury.

TRX straps allow access to a variety of exercises, but most lack quality. Their difficulty lies in the instability inherent in the execution - a deterrent to the acquisition of strength. Working muscles spend most of their time and energy *balancing* the body and *perfecting* the new skill which detracts from what should be the goal - strength gain. And worse: Trainers and trainees often confuse the two. As things get easier with TRX movements, everyone assumes they are getting stronger when the bulk of improvement relates to skill. Worse yet: When the *balance* component of some exercises is combined with an inverted delivery of resistance to the muscles, the risk of injury is elevated as muscle/joint systems reach their extension limits. In other words, the same criticism hurled at the Nautilus cam when it first appeared (that the resistance *felt* too heavy when muscles reached a position of full stretch), has been conveniently re-packaged. The only difference is the addition of a free and dangerous prize – instability.

TRX, in a nutshell:

- Bodyweight is a poor source of resistance (if you have a choice).
- Resistance is inadequately applied to muscles throughout the range of motion.
- The skills acquired through TRX use do *not* transfer to other activities, including golf.

Therefore, if you wish to learn a variety of useless skills (*unrelated to golf*) that produce minimal strength gains and expose muscles to dangerous forces in the process, try TRX. As your suspension skills improve, your body may adapt and avoid injury. But, if you choose TRX training to improve golf, look elsewhere. There are better choices.

Pilates

Pilates is movement-oriented exercise that believes in a strong central foundation as the key to strength and movement. It advocates that energy for exercise is generated from the center of the body outward; that strength in the muscles of the *core* is crucial to movement dynamics; that movement patterns are improved by emphasizing control through proper form and breathing; that movement should be fluid; and that every movement has a purpose related to a greater whole.

The claimed benefits of participation include increased strength, flexibility, cardiovascular ability (when exercises are performed with little or no rest between), body composition and protection from injury.

Does the shoe fit for golf?

Despite the fact that some muscle groups trained via Pilates are rarely exercised by traditional means, the emphasis on strengthening *core* muscles often ignores the larger, stronger muscles that produce power in the golf swing. The counter: Large muscle groups derive their strength and movement control from the center of the body, because stability in the core muscles always *precedes* movement. It does. Every time movement occurs, the body braces itself for the effort by checking its parameters of balance and stability. I have no qualms about strengthening any muscle in the body (because most are involved in golf), but I object to the emphasis on small (*versus* large) muscle groups – the equivalent of training only forearms for golf. And I've seen that.

Strengthening major muscle groups through Pilates is limited by the tools employed. Isolated, direct and full-range exercise is impossible with the equipment in general use - the Cadillac® and the Reformer.® Pilates classes performed on mats and without equipment rely on body weight as resistance – a poor alternative. And - as confirmed on Hole #11 - the most important muscles of the core *cannot* be strengthened by Pilates exercise. Ninety seconds on the MedX Lumbar Extension machine would do more to strengthen the muscles that extend the spine than months of Pilates training.

The strength benefits of Pilates are also limited by the absence of high levels of intensity. The reported claims of *a difficult workout* are more likely related to the difficulty of learning a new skill than exercising muscles to fatigue.

The commercial claim that Pilates leaves you *refreshed, relaxed and rejuvenated*, says it all. When the strength component of an exercise is under-emphasized, or absent, it's time to look elsewhere:

> *This is not to suggest that some strengthening and conditioning does not take place, but that the extent to which this occurs is far more modest than the industry believes and with far better methods available to enhance an individual's physical function.*[1]

To add:

- The failure to meaningfully strengthen the major muscle groups of the body severely limits the degree of claimed cardiovascular benefit, body-composition change and protection from injury.
- Pilates does not create *long, lean muscles* as advertized. The length of a muscle is genetically determined and increases only as a momentary adaptation to movement.
- The core or 'powerhouse' is powerful imagery, but not true. Energy for exercise is generated by the muscle(s) initiating the movement, not necessarily from the center of the body.

- Specific breathing patterns during exercise are not as important as advertised. Your body senses a need and responds. Breathing does not increase results, but its lack may prevent them.
- Fluid movement during the performance of Pilates exercise has more to do with safety than function. It will *not* smooth out your golf swing.
- Pilates is sustained by a powerful marketing arm. Serious golfers can make better use of their time.

Kettlebell Workouts

Ten years ago I returned to my place of birth, Welland, Ontario to see what remained of a once-thriving steel town along the banks of the famous canal that linked Lake Erie to Lake Ontario. Not much. The steel industry had folded, Canada's only John Deere® plant had closed, and the downtown bridges that fascinated me as a boy were dysfunctional. The canal had been replaced by a broader channel that bypassed the city. The telephone directory led me to the only gym in town, the *Galaxy 2000* located in a two-story building formerly occupied by Switson Industries, a small-parts manufacturing firm in the heart of the industrial zone. It was there that I got my first glimpse of kettlebells.

Steps beyond the reception, in a dim corner of a museum-quality room sat what appeared to be a display of cannonballs from the war of 1812-14. A pair of spheres joined by a rusty handle represented a dumbbell. A single sphere - with an off-centered handle - was called a kettlebell. The latter has made a timely comeback in multi-color and been linked, as you might have guessed, to golf performance.

My first glimpse of their use was less impressive - people swinging weights in what I considered *bad form*. Apparently, that's what they do with kettlebells.

Kettlebell handles are positioned beyond the implement's center of gravity which allows limbs to travel with less control through their range of motion. The momentum created during use may force joints and muscles to exceed a safe range of motion, which is why kettlebell trainers go to great lengths to establish a safe starting position from which to work. They must. And, they go to great lengths to limit the range of motion - a practice that increases safety, but does nothing for flexibility.

Specialists claim three benefits from their use: increased strength, power and cardiovascular condition. With proper use, the strength claims equal those of free-weights – but proper use is rare. *Swinging* weights with momentum does *not* build strength as effectively as *lifting* weights. And, demonstrating power in the gym has nothing to do with its development or application on the field.

A recent study[2] at California State University compared the effectiveness of kettlebell exercises to traditional weight-lifting exercises. Specifically, it compared the kettlebell swing, accelerated squat and 'goblet' squat to the traditional high dead-lift, power clean and back squat. Following six weeks of exercise with thirty untrained subjects, they measured strength and power. Gains were similar in the vertical jump (a measure of power), but different in regard to strength: The barbell group increased by 13.6 percent, the kettlebell group by 4.5 percent. The difference was attributed to the increased momentum with kettlebell use.

Compare the results to that of Project Total Conditioning (Hole #13), where the implementation of superior tools, proper supervision, high levels of intensity and strict form proved that strength and power can be obtained safely and more effectively through the use of *slow and controlled* movements.

The use of compound, multi-joint exercises - and brief rest between movements - makes kettlebell training a popular choice for cardiovascular benefits. Is it a good one?

Research[3] at Truman State University in Missouri compared a ten-minute kettlebell swing routine (thirty-five seconds of swinging, alternated with twenty-five seconds of rest) to a ten-minute treadmill run. They kept the effort as constant as they could by matching the 'perceived effort' of the two activities, specifically adjusting the speed of the treadmill to match the effort perceived by the kettlebell workout. The kettlebell routine maintained heart rates above 85 percent of maximum values, enough to stimulate change. But, despite the fact that subjects had to continually increase the speed of the treadmill to keep up with the effort level of the kettlebell workout, the treadmill burned more calories and consumed more oxygen (39 percent versus 25 percent). The study described the aerobic effect of kettlebell training as *decent*, but it did not stack up to traditional training.

Of greatest concern, kettlebell training pushes safety to its limits.

In a University of Waterloo study[4] (Waterloo, Ontario), Stuart McGill reported that kettlebell training exposed spinal vertebrae to more lateral than compression force – a supposed plus compared to a deadlift exercise. Praise for the kettlebell swing was clouded by the fact that not all low backs tolerated the movement and that there was greater activation of glute *versus* lumbar muscles, something the Nautilus inventor believed was a potential cause of back problems. The study stressed the importance of form and warned certain back conditions to avoid kettlebell swings. I'd strengthen my back through MedX lumbar exercise before any attempt.

If strength is the major reason to perform exercise for golf - as it should be - you might put kettlebell training on the back burner.

Vibration Training

Vibration training evolved from the former Soviet Union space program as an attempt to expose cosmonauts to exercise in a non-gravity environment. Its theory evolves from the formula: *Force = Mass x Acceleration*. Traditional strength training increases the resistance (mass) to augment force output. Vibration training claims to affect the acceleration component by increasing the earth's gravitational pull (from one to as much as 1.8 G's). Accordingly, vibrating muscles during exercise increases force requirements and fiber recruitment which, in turn, magnifies and accelerates strength gains.

Research suggests otherwise. In a recent review of literature, the studies cited demonstrated *no* significant difference in strength gains between performing exercise *with* or *without* vibration: research on squats by B. Ronnestad, 2004 and 2009; research on dynamic biceps curls by K. Moran, 2007; research on knee extensions by J. Luo, 2008; and a review of literature by Nordlund and Thorstensson, 2007. *"The research to date,"* concluded the review, *"appears not to support the use of VT (vibration training) for improving strength to a greater extent than resistance training alone."* [5]

Power Plate©, the self-proclaimed leader in vibration technology, points to the number of professional teams and athletes using their technology. Someone bites on a sales pitch, and *voilà*, a platform magically appears in your facility. Without knowing much about it, everyone jumps on board and it's a done deal. If vibration training accelerated strength gains to the extent claimed, every bodybuilder in the world would be on it. Either it doesn't work as claimed, or bodybuilders are smarter than given credit for. My guess is the former. When no one really knows what occurs from a strength perspective with vibration, it's easy to nod your head – or nod off.

Vibration applied to working muscles raises as many questions as answers.

One: In theory, vibration creates corporal instability which is then countered by muscle contraction to recreate a homeostatic state. This, in part, is the claim experts make about vibration's ability to recruit a greater number of muscle fibers during exercise. If your purpose, however, is to strengthen biceps on a Power Plate by performing a standing curl with a barbell, why vibrate your entire body? Whole-body vibration sends a signal to distribute blood *throughout* the body as a perceived need. You want the majority of that distribution - if not all - directed to your biceps. I was always reminded to relax muscles that were *not* working during exercise.

Two: Vibration platforms have attached cords that add a variety of exercises to the menu. The vibration transmitted through the cords is so muted, however, that the manufacturer suggests options to improve its quality: The cord can be adjusted to a position that creates more friction as it exits the machine; *or* can be pulled at a faster speed which increases friction and provides a sensation of greater resistance. More than the tool should be questioned when *bad* form (faster movement is always a step in the wrong direction) is recommended to improve results. In any case, the increase in resistance provided by the cords working *at their best* is inadequate to stimulate the desired result.

Vibration websites reference more than 180 studies that demonstrate the positive effect of their product on a multitude of training variables beyond strength. Some claims are substantiated.

The Power Plate is effective for flexibility. Vibration restrains sensors that inhibit muscles from reaching length limits, thereby allowing a greater stretch. Cardiovascular claims are also valid if exercise is performed with limited rest between efforts - a result produced by *any* form of exercise.

Increases in bone density are poor with vibration training because strength gains are poor. The Power Plate flagship study (published in *The Journal of Bone and Mineral Research*, 2004) boasts a 1.5 percent increase in *bone density* over a twenty-four-week training period. According to Margaret Martin, a physical therapist from Ottawa who reviewed the study, *"The reason the Power Plate group showed an increase in hip area bone density over the study period – compared to the other groups – was not due to the benefits of the PPVP (Power Plate Vibration Platform). It was a result of the exercise program that they followed."*[6] The Power Plate group performed progressive weight-bearing exercises; the traditional-trained group performed non-progressive, non-weight-bearing endurance (aerobic) exercises – the type that has yet to produce a positive outcome in reference to bone density.

Nonetheless, the reported 1.5 percent increase in bone density is dismal. Many studies (Pollock, 1992; Menkes, 1993; Braith and others, 1996) demonstrate greater increases using traditional equipment and strength-training methods.

Another claim (from the Power Plate website) is fantasy:

> *Acceleration training on a Power Plate stimulates fast-twitch muscle fibers and athletes who use Power Plate machines over time experience a dramatic increase in explosive strength, motor learning, muscular endurance and overall agility.*

Dream on. Fast-twitch muscle fibers are activated by intensity, and the catalytic effect of vibration does not appear to trigger the claimed response. Explosive strength is a product of genetic endowment, muscle strength and body-fat levels, and is not accelerated by the training methods suggested. Motor learning cannot increase with vibration on a Power Plate because of the laws governing specificity and transfer established on Hole #2. If strength gains are poor, local muscle endurance gains are equally poor. And finally, agility is genetically determined, and not subject to change.

If vibration training works as well as claimed, why not vibrate a superior form of resistance - a Nautilus machine? Given time, somebody will.

Arthur Jones applauded any innovation that made exercise more productive. *"Design it, build it, strap it on your back and head off down the runway,"* he said, *"then it will either fly or it won't; but until you try it, you will never know for sure."*

Last I heard, vibration training's self-proclaimed leader filed for financial restructure. Guess it didn't fly.

Cross-Training

Cross-training systems (P90X®, CrossFit®, Extreme Training®, Insanity® Training, etc.) are based upon two cornerstones of Nautilus training in the 1970's: intensity and minimal rest between efforts. Both increase the overall quality of the stimulus, but that's where the similarity ends.

Nautilus training was efficient. The full-body workout of Miami-Dolphin running-back, Mercury Morris, outlined in Ellington Darden's, *Strength Training Principles,* 1977, was clocked at thirteen minutes and six seconds. The average time between exercises was thirteen seconds, which included securing seat belts.

In contrast, some cross-training programs insist on an hour or more of exercise each day, five or six days a week, and rationalize their stance by performing *different* activities, or by training distinct muscle groups each day. The weight of scientific evidence suggests that strength training - or any form of strenuous physical activity - performed on consecutive days interferes with systemic recovery.

Arthur Jones often confronted bodybuilders who trained everyday *in parts* with the following: *"Sleep tonight with your left eye open, tomorrow night with your right, and tell me how you do.*" By the time it registered, he was off to the next prototype.

My first view of cross-training occurred in the Lake Toxaway Country Club Fitness Center (NC) in 2008. Three guests asked if we had a skipping rope, which we did not. So, they traveled to a local hardware store, returned and promptly downloaded a *CrossFit* workout from the internet.

I've seen idiots in my day, but this youthful trio took the cake. Curly, Larry and Moe jumped around like kangaroos for twenty minutes, eliminating any need of vibration. The routine - laden with impact and potential injury - was an orthopedic dream.

Cross-training's application to golf relates to the fact that golf is a *power* sport, and that cross-training has an affinity for *power* exercises (explosive movements). Beware. Intensity, not speed of movement, governs muscle fiber recruitment, as determined by research:

"The evidence suggests that individuals should be encouraged to train to momentary muscular failure, as this appears to maximize muscle-fiber recruitment and, according to most of the research to date, will maximize gains in strength and power."[7]

To the surprise and dismay of many, strength, power and momentary muscle failure can be safely acquired by the performance of slow, controlled movements. In contrast, the adherence to 'explosive' speed and impact may one day prevent you from moving at all.

The intensity of cross-training can elicit a cardiovascular response and improve body composition, but expect a loss in flexibility unless a stretching protocol is added. Workouts are laden with multi-joint exercises performed through an incomplete range of motion.

The PGA Tour continues to promote their athletes as super-talented in activities other than golf, while many experts believe that a cross-trained athlete is a better athlete. Research and logic disagree. From a skill perspective, the *only* way to improve in a sport is to practice the sport, not a dozen other activities. From a fitness viewpoint, the physical condition gained by playing a sport may possess a degree of specificity, but participation in another activity – any activity - that increases strength, cardiovascular capacity or flexibility may benefit the target activity.

I wouldn't give cross-training a glance. Golfers can get more fit in less time, in a safer manner.

References

1. Robert Morrison, "Pilates: The Irrefutable Truth," *Synergy* (IART publication, 2007).
2. W.H. Otto et al., "Effects of Weightlifting vs. Kettlebell Training on Vertical Jump, Strength, and Body Composition," *Journal of Strength and Conditioning Research* 26, no. 5 (2012), 1199.
3. Caleb Hulsey et al., "Comparison of Kettlebell Swings and Treadmill Running at Equivalent Rating of Perceived Exertion Values," *Journal of Strength and Conditioning Research* 26 (2012), 1203.
4. Stuart McGill and L.W. Marshall, "Kettlebell Swing, Snatch, and Bottoms-up Carry: Back and Hip Muscle Activation Motion, and Low Back Loads," *Journal of Strength and Conditioning Research* 26, no. 1 (2012), 16.
5. M.M. Nordlund and A. Thorstensson, "Strength Training Effects of Whole-Body Vibration?" *Scandinavian Journal of Medicine and Science in Sports* 17, no. 1 (2007), 12.
6. Margaret Martin, "Will the Power Plate Alone Increase Bone Density?" *melioguide*, http://www.melioguide.com/osteoporosis-exercise-equipment/will-the-power-plate-alone-increase-bone-density/
7. James Fisher et al., "Evidence-Based Resistance Training Recommendations," *Medicina Sportiva* 15, no. 3 (2011), 147.

Hole #17: 420 Yards, Par 4

THE HOME STRETCH

In 1975, Bob Anderson published a book that introduced readers to the joy and benefits of movement. Five years later, a revised edition of *Stretching* became an international best-seller. In 2000, he upgraded his effort to include a greater variety of stretches, plus different tools and techniques to improve the quality of the experience.

Of particular note (in all editions) was a section on stretching for popular activities and sports, including golf. I followed Anderson's recommendations for thirty years and enjoyed some of the claimed benefits:

Stretching ...

- Reduces muscle tension and makes the body feel more relaxed.
- Helps coordination by allowing for freer and easier movement.
- Increases range of motion.
- Helps prevent injuries such as muscle strains (a strong and flexible pre-stretched muscle resists stress better than a strong, stiff and un-stretched muscle).
- Has preparatory value - signals muscles that they are about to be used.
- Helps maintain your current level of flexibility.
- Develops body awareness, by focusing on targeted muscles and the process.
- Helps loosen the mind's control of the body to allow the body to move for its own sake, rather than for competition or ego.
- Feels good.

Not everyone agrees.

John Little, author of *The Max Golf Workout,* believes that claims of increased range of motion (short-term) and flexibility (long-term) are temporary. Like a rubber band, he asserts, the muscle gradually returns to its original state. This explains the need to engage in stretching activities on a regular (perhaps daily) basis, and supports Anderson's claim that stretching can *maintain* a current level of flexibility. Little also believes that metabolic activity (muscle contraction, not elongation) is the key to pre-game activity, including golf. Anderson agrees. The latest edition of his book offers warm-up suggestions *before* stretching for vigorous physical activities. And, it is common knowledge that stretching a muscle does not prevent injury to the degree that strengthening can.

Both authors discuss the topic from distinct perspectives: Little, a hard-core strength enthusiast influenced by Arthur Jones; and Anderson, an expert in stretching. They are not far apart. Muscle strength is the key to generating and resisting force in the golf swing. It produces the motion of the swing, and protects the body from injury. Flexibility plays a secondary role: It facilitates movement through a greater range of motion.

The pre-golf warm-up in *The Max Golf Workout* consists of several practice swings on the tee, or hitting a few practice balls. Little's assumption is that flexibility has already been addressed through the proper use of Nautilus machines during a workout, a notion I support. Anderson's warm up consists of brief stretching (5-10 minutes) *before* play or practice. I've done that as well - and arrive at no conclusion.

Stretching *before* play has provided the following personal benefits (from the list above):

- Reduces muscle tension and makes the body feel more relaxed.
- Has preparatory value - signals muscles that they are about to be used.
- Feels good.

The benefits are both physiological and psychological - and the psychological plays a huge role in golf. If you *feel* ready to play, you might *be* ready. I don't know how many times I've rushed to the first tee without preparation or warm-up wondering where my ball will finish, or how I might play. The ritual of performing a pre-game routine, *any* routine, does not guarantee good play - but it does provide psychological comfort, even among the elite.

The pre-game routine of Spain's Miguel Angel Jimenez, for example, has captured media attention from the time he began the bizarre ritual. One announcer commented, *"What does* that *have to do with golf?"* It may have nothing to do with golf, but that's not the point. Habits have great personal value – and golfers are a superstitious lot.

With that in mind, let's review stretching principles and a brief, full-body stretch routine to assist golfers on and off the course.

Stretching Principles (from Bob Anderson's, *Stretching*)

- Focus attention on a relaxed, sustained stretch in the targeted muscle(s).
- Slowly move to an *easy stretch* position - a degree of tension that feels comfortable (not forced) - and hold it for 10-15 seconds.
- When the tension subsides, move slowly into a *developmental stretch* position (a fraction of an inch further until another mild stretch is felt). Hold it, again, for 10-15 seconds.
- If the tension of either stretch position does not diminish, ease off slightly.
- Breathe slow and relaxed. Exhale as you move into a stretch position.
- *Do not bounce* when moving toward, or after assuming, a position of stretch.

Golf Stretches on Course

The following stretches (in order) can be performed on the course *before* or *after* golf. Stretches performed with the assistance of a golf club are marked with an asterisk (*). Those performed using a golf cart as a prop are indicated by a double asterisk (**).

1. **Overhead Reach** (Shoulders, Upper Back and Arms)

- Interlace your fingers (palms up) above your head and push your arms up and slightly back. Hold for *fifteen seconds.*

  * Same as above using a golf club with hands held close together in the middle of the shaft.

  ** Grasp the roof of a cart with both hands. Bend your knees slightly and allow your torso to sag toward the ground. Relax your head and neck.

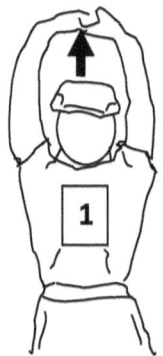 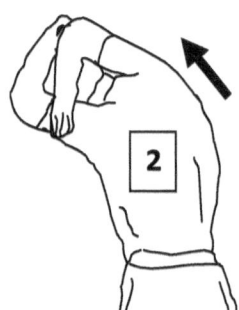

Variations include:

Overhead Reach with Twist

- From the overhead reach position, and without moving your feet, twist your head and shoulders to the right. Hold for *ten seconds.* Repeat to the left.

  ** Grasping the roof of a golf cart, cross your right hand about twelve inches over the left and turn your shoulders and head to the right. Repeat by crossing your left hand over the right, and turning to the left.

2. **Side-Bend** (Shoulders and Upper Back)

    *   With arms above your head, grasp your opposite elbow and gently pull it behind your head as you bend from the hips to the same side. Keep your knees slightly bent. Hold for *ten seconds* on each side.

        * Place your hands shoulder-width apart on the club. Gently pull on the club to the right as you bend in that direction. Repeat to the left.

        ** Stand with your left shoulder facing the side of a cart. Reach your right hand over your head and grasp the cart roof as you bend from the hips. Repeat with your left arm.

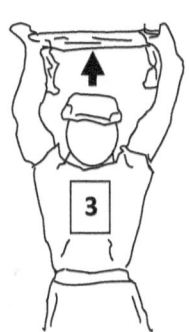 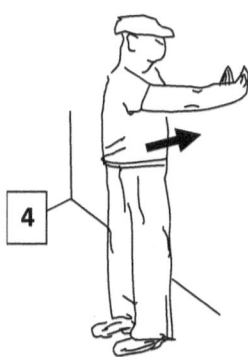

3. **Behind-Head Reach** (Shoulders, Chest and Arms)

    *   Grab a towel at both ends so you can move it, with straight arms, up and over your head, and down behind your back. If the movement is difficult, use a wider grip. Hold for *fifteen seconds*.
        (This stretch can be tough on shoulders, so proceed accordingly)

        * Same as above but separate your hands to the ends of the club and narrow the width of the grip as you progress.

Variations include:

Behind-Head Reach with Outward Pull

- Gently pull outward on the ends of the towel or club. Hold for *fifteen seconds.*

4. **Trunk Rotation** (Upper/Middle Back and Spine)

- Stand 12-24 inches from a wall (or imaginary wall) with your back to it, feet shoulder-width apart and toes pointed straight forward. Without allowing your feet to move, slowly turn to the right and touch the wall at shoulder height. Hold for *10-15 seconds.* Repeat to the left.

   * Hold a club waist-high with a shoulder-width grip and arms extended. Turn to your right trying to reach a position in which the shaft is parallel to your toe line, but behind you. Repeat to the left.

   ** Use the cart as your wall.

5. **Calf Stretch** (Calves and Lower Leg)

- Stand 2-3 feet from a wall or solid support and lean on the support with your hands or forearms.

Step forward with one leg (bent) and straighten the rear leg. Keeping your low back flat, move your hips forward and downward without raising the heel of the rear leg off the floor. Keep toes pointing straight forward and hold for *thirty seconds* with each leg.

   * Use a golf club as your base of support (as you would a cane).

   ** Use a golf cart as your wall.

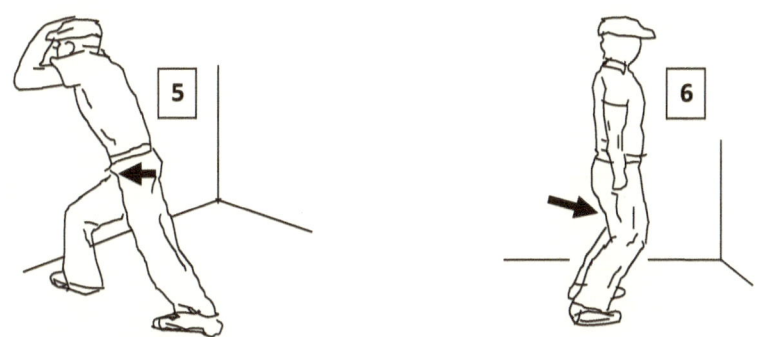

6. **Soleus Stretch** (Soleus and Lower Leg)

- Stand straight and bend slightly at the knee without allowing your heels to leave the floor. Now, shift your hips forward and bend your knees a little more (while maintaining heel contact). Hold for *twenty seconds.*

7. **Standing Hamstring Stretch** (Hamstrings, Hips and Low Back)

- With your knees slightly bent and feet shoulder-width apart, slowly bend forward from the hips and reach toward the ground. Keep your arms and neck relaxed. Focus on the stretch in the back of your legs. Hold for *twenty seconds.*

  * Same as above holding a golf club with a shoulder-width grip.

  ** Place your extended right leg on a cart at gas-pedal height. With your toe turned up and knee slightly bent, slowly reach toward your right foot (leading with hips). Repeat with left leg.

Variations include:

Standing Hamstring Stretch with Twist *

- From the stretch position, slowly turn your torso to the left, 90° - rest the golf-club shaft on the outside of your left ankle and perpendicular to your toe line. Hold for *ten seconds*. Repeat to the right.

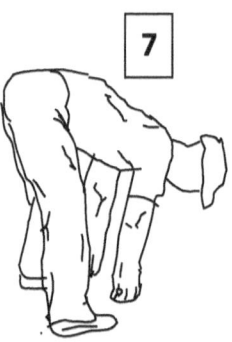 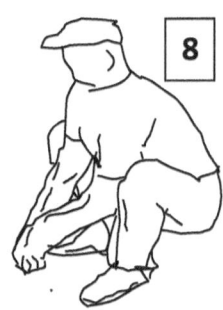

8. Deep Squat (Low Back, Front Thighs and Hips)

Squat down with your feet flat on the ground and toes pointed out slightly. Keep knees outside of shoulders and directly above feet. Hold for *thirty seconds*.

Variations include:

Deep Squat with Groin Stretch

- During the deep squat, push your knees gently outward with your elbows. Hold for *ten seconds*.

Deep Squat with Reach

- Before standing up, reach forward toward the ground ahead. Hold for *ten seconds*.

   * *Reach forward with a club held by both hands.*

Note: Stretches 9 through 11 require contact with the ground. Restrict their use to a clean floor or carpet at home.

9. **Seated Groin Stretch** (Inner Thigh and Lower Back)

- Sit on the floor and unite the soles of your feet in front of you. Hold your toes together and pull yourself forward from the hips with a straight back. Hold for *thirty seconds*.

Variations include:

Seated Groin Stretch with Knee Push

- During the seated groin stretch, push your knees gently outward by using elbows or hands. Hold for *fifteen seconds*.

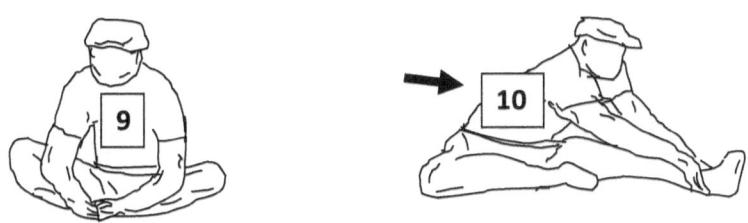

10. **Seated Hamstring Stretch** (Hamstrings and Low Back)

- From the seated groin stretch position (Stretch #9, above), extend your left leg to the side while the right leg remains bent in front (right sole touching the inside of your left thigh). Slowly bend forward from the hips and reach toward the left leg with both hands. If difficult, slightly bend the extended knee. Hold for *thirty seconds*. Repeat with right leg extended.

11. **Forearm Stretch** (Forearm and Biceps)

- Assume an *all-fours* position on the floor. Invert your hands so that fingers point toward your knees, palms down, thumbs out. Keep your head in line with your torso. *Slowly* and *slightly*, shift your torso toward your heels without losing hand contact. Hold for *20 seconds*.

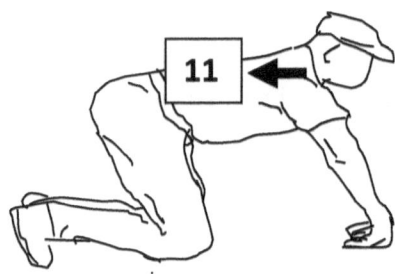

The entire routine (Stretches 1-11) requires approximately six minutes, and yields best results when performed *after* golf.

A competent instructor can teach you how to stretch; a fitness trainer can teach you how to get the most from strength training; and a golf professional can teach you how to best refine your skills. There is a side to golf, however, that can't be taught - can only be learned. The final hole takes you on a brief journey through a golfer's mind, the ultimate frontier in sports performance.

Hole #18: 321 Yards, Par 4

FROM THE NECK UP

"Golf is an easy game, until you start to care."
Charlie Rymer, The Golf Channel

B y the time you reach the final hole, you should know where you stand for the day. If good, you want to finish strong - preserve your accomplishments to that point; if not, you want to finish. And when something's on the line – a bet, a best score, a championship – the pressure is amplified. *"Golf is an easy game, until you start to care"* rings true, and care starts from the neck up. Suddenly the putt or wager takes on greater significance, or the moment reflects years of input - you can't let yourself or your partner(s) down. The anxiety of performing *on call* can make the physical preparation for golf feel like a walk in the park.

It escapes no one.

The Sunday I watched Moe Norman tee off in the Canadian Open at St. Georges in Toronto, 1968 (referenced on Hole #13) had a higher calling. George Knudson, *The Great Canadian Hope*, was tied for the lead with New Zealand's Bob Charles entering the final round of a tournament that a Canadian had not won since Pat Fletcher in 1954. Hope was high. Knudson had already won two events on the PGA Tour that season, scored a hole-in-one during the second round, and tied the course record of sixty-four in the third. But the field was bunched. Six players were one shot behind; four others, two back.

Knudson was paired with Tommy Aaron and Charlie Sifford in the final group, preceded by Casper, Nicklaus and Charles. The balance and rhythm of both Aaron and Knudson remain etched in my memory. Knudson fashioned his swing after Ben Hogan, and it showed. He hit every green on the front nine and was not outside of twenty feet. His stellar play, however, did not pay off: George couldn't putt. On the par-three sixth, a 210-yard gem with a forced carry to a small green, he hit a long iron four feet above the hole and three putted. His two-over-par seventy-three reflected a burden he could not shoulder. In the end, Bob Charles edged out Jack Nicklaus by a single stroke.

In a similar fashion, my grit was put to the test on the final tee at the Porter Cup in 1973. The eighteenth hole was a mid-length par-three surrounded by bunkers. I needed a birdie to qualify. My tee shot finished twelve feet right of the cup, a putt I read from every angle. The pressure of the moment took me out of my routine, and by surprise. When the putt slipped by, it felt as if someone had sucked the air from the planet. But there was good news: I didn't need the putt after all. My 74-72, the *"highest qualifying score in the history of the tournament,"* according to one official, made the final spot, and reminded me of a slice of wisdom I heard along the way: *"Why worry? You might worry about the wrong thing."* I celebrated with a lengthy run.

Golf's anxious moments are fostered between the ears. The mind creates problems that lead to poor decisions, to fear and doubt. It partners with your current status and plays games with your thought process, often establishing the voice you hear as you stand over your next effort: *Keep your head steady; Don't pull this putt like you did the last one; Swing through the ball.* Golfers talk to themselves all the time, mumbling instructions internally and externally both before and after the fact. The mind is easily distracted, and the less information it handles, the better.

The mental input and response during play is heightened by the following:

- The challenge of the course (a narrow fairway, water hazard or out-of-bounds).
- The immediate circumstance (a bet, close match or needed putt).
- Time between efforts – time to ponder the consequences of failure or success.

Historically, the game has teased players with the notion that they once did - and still can - hit a perfect shot. The first time you looked up and saw the ball sail straight to your target, it was miraculous. You didn't know how it happened, but you were hooked. Those who *make it happen* more frequently have honed their skills to a higher level and make it appear effortless. They have simplified the process, and no longer step on their own toes.

Moe Norman was the perfect example of simplicity. He never took a lesson or a practice swing – but groomed his skills by hitting millions of balls. During an exhibition I witnessed in the 1990's, someone asked, *"Hey Moe, when was the last time you hit a shot off line."* He hesitated a few seconds and replied, *"1963."* Everyone laughed, but he was serious. I recently watched a one-hour video of Moe hitting shots that he described as either *"Perfect,"* or *"As pure as the driven snow"* – shot after shot after shot. His word choice was not habit, but descriptive. I then turned to a televised PGA Tour event and saw nothing but players leaning side to side, slumping heads, tapping clubs and begging golf balls – shot after shot after shot. The contrast was vivid.

Perfect was not an opinion with Moe Norman: He simply did not hit a ball off-line. If he had played on the PGA Tour (there were reasons he did not), peers would have stopped to watch, as they did with Ben Hogan. After he retired from competition, Moe often appeared at the practice tee of the Canadian Open, and - as ritual had it - was invited by a current player to *"hit a few."* With street shoes and a borrowed club, Moe rifled ball after ball, often out of divots, straight down the range. One by one, players gathered to witness something to which they could only aspire. As Hall-of-Fame teaching professional Craig Shankland (a friend of Moe's for twenty years) described, *"Watching him hit balls was riveting. You could not believe how good it was, time after time."*

To many, he was the prince of golf; to others, a diversion. Moe's swing and mannerisms were different. *"People laughed at me,"* he said, *"because I made it look so easy."*

Lorne Rubenstein, a Canadian author who followed Norman's career, believed he knew why:

> *Moe turned golf into a reaction sport rather than a creation sport. He played golf as if it were hockey or baseball; he was reacting rather than initiating a motion. Moe looked at the target, assimilated all*

the information he needed, and swung immediately: his swing was his reaction. All golfers want to play the game without thinking. His nature compelled him to play that way.[1]

Moe Norman did everything quickly - walk, swing, putt and talk. *"Winners play golf automatically,"* he said. *"Winners see what they want. Losers see what they don't want. Don't let the game eat you. You eat the game. He* (Moe) *defined golf as* 'hitting an object to a defined target area with the least amount of effort and an alert attitude of indifference.' *Every golfer should let himself play, not make himself play."*[2]

According to Rubenstein, quick mannerisms played to his advantage. *"Moe played outside time because he took no time. He thereby neutralized the psychological complexities of the game, all part of turning it into a reaction sport."*

The concept of *automatic* is nothing new. In an article, '*The Psychology of Golf,*' published in the *North American Review* (1897), Dr. Louis Robinson stated:

> *It is essential to give one's whole self to each state of the game if anything like success is to be hoped for. But one must do it in a kind of passive and animal fashion, committing the business as it were to that sub-agent of the will who is in charge of the automatic department. Any attempt to bring the conscious will into play, as one is often tempted to do after a series of exasperating failures, at once sets the automatic department on strike.*[3]

I played my best golf when I arrived at the top of my backswing *before* I realized I was ready. My effort was a far cry from the reactionary ease of Moe Norman, but it embraced minimal thought: Take in the landscape, and trust your homework.

… easier said than done.

Tennis professional, Timothy Gallway recognized the role of the mind in sports performance and sought to diminish its influence in a practical way. His book, *The Inner Game of Tennis*, revealed a method of distracting the mind by focusing on an easy-to-do, related idea. The majority of beginners, he found, struggled with proper footwork, and traditional teaching only complicated the process. Gallway had his students focus on two events: The moment the ball bounced in front of them, they said - to themselves or aloud – "*Bounce;*" and the moment the racquet struck the ball, "*Hit.*" The focus on *Bounce-Hit* had an immediate effect on footwork. Gallway explained the phenomenon as eliminating mind clutter to allow the body to do what it already can. He developed techniques that applied to other aspects of tennis, and then turned his attention to golf.

Time factors were different in golf. Tennis involved reacting to an object; golf involved initiating the action. Through trial and error, the *Bounce-Hit* of tennis became the *Back-Hit* of golf. The moment the club reached its backswing apex, you said, "*Back,*" and the instant the club contacted the ball, "*Hit.*"

I first read Gallway's sequel, *The Inner Game of Golf,* in Venezuela. At the time, I hadn't played for seven years, but had recently joined a club. The *Back-Hit* concept seemed as foreign as my return, but I had nothing to lose. One day, on the par-three 10th hole at Lagunita Country Club in El Hatillo, I decided to focus on the *time factors* of golf. *When* the club reached the top of my swing, I said "*Back,*" and *when* it struck the ball, I said "*Hit.*" I would have bet my life on a gentle fade (a left-to-right ball flight) with a three iron – but my effort was greeted by a pleasant surprise, a gentle draw (a right-to-left ball flight). Not convinced I had performed the mental exercise properly, I hit the same club from the fifteenth fairway and witnessed a similar result. I don't know how it happened - or how it could - but I devoured the book that evening and have since used its techniques to self-correct.

The secret was not *Back-Hit* per se. The related focus on the *when* distracted the back-seat driver within – *left shoulder under the chin, grip pressure, weight shift, butt out, trees left, finish in balance.* My body knew how to hit a perfect shot - I had to get out of its way. The experience mimicked 2014 US Open champion, Martin Kaymer's comment at Pinehurst in a post-play interview, "*I never really advanced much this year until I started getting out of my own way.*"

Roger Bannister took up running because he did not excel at sports that involved the use of a ball. In light of his experience on the track, he knew the mental side of golf:

> *All sporting events are more mental than physical. You have to train the physical aspects for years. But eventually, even in the more complex movements, which have my respect, those who can pitch and bat or play golf and so on, the basis of it is laid down in the brain and the real question is whether the brain can be allowed to do its bit without being interfered with by psychological factors. The other aspect of the brain is that it must be positive. I suppose these two are connected. But the brain has to have some overall image of what is being achieved.*[4]

Moe Norman established that image with a quick glance to his target.

Ignorance is Bliss

I often played golf courses better the first time than the second or third: I didn't know where the hazards were. The fifteenth hole at Prestwick Golf Club in Scotland was a perfect example. It featured large mounds that lined both sides of an elevated fairway hidden beyond. Its length – 325 yards - appeared benign. I nonchalantly hit a tee shot between the mounds and tossed the bag over my shoulder. When I reached the top of the incline, I spotted my ball - in the fairway - surrounded by the deepest pit-bunkers I'd ever seen. If I had known they were there, I'd still be there.

Playing golf with beginners taught me the same – they fail to comprehend degree of difficulty. I once played with a novice who faced a thirty-yard shot to a pin tucked behind a bunker. I could have hit a bucket of balls and never gotten within fifteen feet of the pin, but what did I know? From a downhill lie in the rough, ball above her feet, she hit to four feet from the hole. It wasn't conventional or pretty, but she pulled it off with staggering innocence: *Here's the ball, there's the hole. And it's my turn.*

As is often the case in golf, the less you know the better.

The Comfort Zone

The mind creates a comfort zone related to expectations. A golfer with a five handicap, for example, would expect to break eighty, but not shoot par. When you play within those parameters, you sleep at night. When you get ahead of yourself - out of your comfort zone - you think and play defensively: *When will it all fall apart? How long will my good fortune last?* On the other hand, you think a slump will never end. The nature of the game makes it impossible to predict an outcome, or how you might handle the process. Playing beyond one's expectations is rare and often occurs *out of the blue.* Few can deal with it.

In 1968, several Lookout Point members - because of their success in the event - urged me to play an invitational tournament at the Norfolk Golf and Country Club, Canada's seventh oldest course, established on a hilly parcel of land in Simcoe, Ontario, in 1895. The nine-hole layout featured two sets of tees, narrow tree-lined fairways, and a generous prize table I was fortunate to visit.

The following year, as defending champion, I came off the front nine at one-under par, one ahead of Lookout's club champion, Bob Jarvis. My strategy on the inward nine was to hit fairways and greens. On the tenth hole, I unexpectedly sunk a thirty-foot uphill birdie putt and scurried to the par-three eleventh where I faced a forty-minute delay. When it was my turn, I sunk a twenty-foot birdie putt that I simply nudged toward the hole without expectations. My approach shot to the elevated twelfth green left a slick fifteen-foot birdie putt with a five-foot break. It, too, went in. Success on three putts I did not intend to hole took me out of my comfort zone. I stumbled home with a winning score of one-under par. More holes, and I wouldn't have made it.

The same occurred during a friendly round in Venezuela with national amateur champion, Henrique Lavié. I played the first five holes of the Lagunita Country Club that day at even par, a good start on a tough course. The sixth was a downhill par four that demanded a tee shot in the fairway. My nine-iron approach to a narrow, slanted green found the cup, which triggered a 2-3-2 stretch (eagle, birdie, birdie) and tightened the noose. A three-putt at the ninth loosened its knot.

I birdied the eleventh and fourteenth holes to, once again, exit my comfort zone. A four-iron approach to the fifteenth green left a simple fifteen-foot putt that took three to negotiate. On the next, I three-putted again from twelve feet above the hole – shades of George Knudson. I stumbled home with a three-under par sixty-seven to tie Henrique – who went on to win the Venezuelan PGA Championship in 1995.

Out of the comfort zone is exactly what it implies – combating heightened nerves and tricks the mind plays during a round of golf. The best players in the game battle the phenomenon every week … and are not always successful.

In 1987, I played in the Venezuelan Amateur Match-Play championship at Izcaragua Country Club (thirty minutes east of Caracas), a venue that hosted the National Amateur Stroke-Play championship the week before. I was unprepared. My tenth place finish in the stroke-play event was my first competitive tournament in fourteen years. It left me seeded thirtieth for the match-play competition, and destined to face the recently crowned champion. That was the good news.

My opponent could do it all. Besides a stellar amateur record on the national scene, Carlos Larrain could hit a golf ball a country mile, and find it. He was also playing his home course. Fortunately, I had played with him a number of times, and enjoyed watching his tee shots tower 60-100 yards beyond mine. In fact, on a par-five hole in a friendly match months before on my home course, I hit the green for the first and only time with a drive and three-wood that ran downwind. Carlos flew his approach over the green with a nine iron.

The upcoming match would be a *matter of time.*

Three holes down after nine, I birdied the eleventh. Two holes later, he missed a six-foot putt that would have left me hanging by chewed finger nails. I somehow made it to the seventeenth tee - proud of my survival. I was two holes down with two to play; in golf terms, *dormie.* To my surprise, Carlos hit an errant approach to the dogleg seventeenth, and lost the hole to par. One hole down and one to play – still a *matter of time.*

The Tennessee Connection

In 2001, Venezuelan Carlos Larrain led the Sugura Viudas Challenge de Espana (his first European Challenge Tour event that year) by one shot after two rounds. During a post-game interview, he credited his success to a recent five-day visit with his American coach, John Elliott, a top teaching-professional at Golf Digest® schools.

In the late 1960's, John Elliott was a member of a highly successful golf team at Austin Peay State University in Clarkesville, Tennessee. My brother, Al, was a member of that team.

The eighteenth hole featured an elevated tee to a tight fairway that prompted a three-iron to safety for most. Carlos hammered his driver down the middle, as he had all day. My approach scooted through the green, as I stepped aside to watch him seal my fate. His lofty sand wedge landed short of the flag but, three bounces later, joined my ball in the rough beyond the green. We both hacked out to four feet, and Carlos missed.

I trudged to the first hole, our nineteenth, in disbelief. It was still a *matter of time*. Carlos hit his tee shot through the fairway into a bunker, knocked it on the green and three-putted from thirty-five feet. My par earned a bevy of high-fives from fellow competitors grateful that the top-seed had been eliminated. Unpredictable? You bet. Carlos could beat me eleven times out of ten – like a drum – all day, any day. Ironically, I was defeated on the last hole by his cousin in the following match.

Without a doubt, my opponent had more to lose than me, but he was a gentleman and a champion. The next year, 1988, Carlos won the Brazilian Open as an amateur. In 1999, he won ten of fifteen professional tournaments in Venezuela (with four second-place finishes) and began a three-year stint on the European Challenge Tour. He recently chaired a committee to organize the new Latin-American version of the PGA Tour. My cap remains off.

Both Henrique Lavié and Carlos Larrain were members of the Venezuelan amateur team that trained in my Nautilus facility in 1986.

Simplicity

Competition in golf comes in three forms: You play an opponent, a course and yourself. The final form is, by far, the most demanding. The mind has plenty of time to sabotage performance. Moe Norman would have none of it. Nor would Lee Trevino: It was one look and hit. Tim Gallway's effort to take on the psychological challenges of the game was one of many books to address golf from the neck up. And the increasing number of tour professionals who add psychological gurus to their entourage has brought the importance of the topic to the forefront. Everyone has a team; every team member has input; and every input has purpose.

While some thrive on the approach of a committee, others, like Nautilus inventor, Arthur Jones, did not. *"A committee,"* he said, *"never solved a damn thing."* Did Ben Hogan or Moe Norman have a team around them? No. At best, players from that era had someone who taught them the game and to whom they could return for help, or they helped each other. No one could afford an entourage, which may have been a blessing.

Too much input clogs the drain. The skill, fitness and psychological aspects of the game can - and should - be simplified. Don't cross your fingers.

Golf professionals continue to introduce new ways to address the skill component of the game, and everyone sees it differently. Theories like *Square-to-Square* and *The Connection* are replaced by *Natural Golf* and *The Stack and Tilt*. Some are aimed at simplifying the process, but the fact remains: The more input to the brain, the less likely the chance of success. How many college superstars have derailed by listening to someone advocating perfection? And what do most pros revert to when they are *off* their game? Grip, stance, ball position, aim and posture - a return to basics generally saves the day.

With the exceptions of Frank Stranahan and Gary Player, there was no fitness component to golf in the old days. It was, *"Put down the cigarettes and beer"* or, *"Pick up the cigarettes and beer,"* and play. Physical preparation for golf has enjoyed a recent explosion with trainers leaping off the back of Corn Flakes® boxes – each with a vision. *Zero* participation has become *more is better*, in some cases, training every day for hours, committing the same errors of novice bodybuilders, and more. Timing and clever marketing has turned serious golfers in the direction of functional training, a can of worms that, among other things, increases mental input.

Your golf instructor tells you to keep weight on the inside of your rear foot during your backswing to prevent head and torso sway; your fitness trainer suggests that your left deltoid needs stretching to make a better backswing turn, that your right hip needs an explosive move towards the target from the top of the swing, and that your right rotator cuff is tight which affects your ability to assume a *tray* position during your backswing; and your psychologist has you performing *monkey slumps* on the tee to stabilize breathing and calm nerves. And worse: They coordinate efforts. How can you excel at - or enjoy - a game you have so complicated?

I don't believe you can, to the degree you should.

When I first joined a club in Caracas, I played once a week, hardly enough to progress – and endured six-hour rounds. One day, I lightened my load by leaving four clubs in the car and broke eighty. From there, I decided to see if I could break eighty with one less club per week. I succeeded with nine, eight, seven, six, five and four clubs on consecutive Sundays. The challenge simplified things, made me work harder, and rekindled my interest in the game.

In a similar context, a female playing partner once asked, *"Why do I have seven clubs? They all go the same distance."* I had no reply.

Keep it simple. Play with *"an alert attitude of indifference."*

References

1. Lorne Rubenstein, *Moe & Me* (Toronto, ON: ECW Press, 2012), 28.
2. Lorne Rubenstein, *Moe & Me* (Toronto, ON: ECW Press), 2012), 63.
3. Louis Robinson, "The Psychology of Golf," *North American Review* 165, no. 493 (1897), 649. http://ebooklibrary.org/eBooks/ WPLBN0002165094-The-North-American-Review--Volume-0165-

Issue-493-December-1897-North-American-review-and-mis-by-University-of-Northern-Iowa.aspx?&Trail=collection&Words=

4. Academy of Achievement, "Sir Roger Bannister Interview," Compilation of two interviews conducted October 27, 2000 (London, England) and June 7, 2002 (Dublin, Ireland), http://www.achievement.org/autodoc/page/ban0int-7.

A WEE NIP

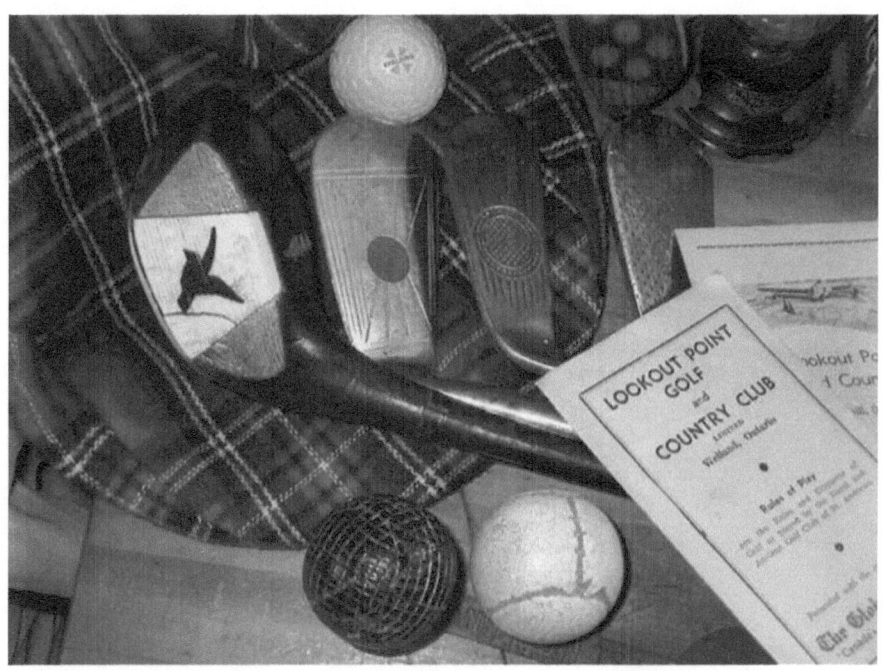

The 19th Hole

HOME AT LAST

The nineteenth hole, an integral part of the Royal and Ancient game, symbolizes a time and place for beverage, camaraderie, review and story-telling. Though many of its tales should remain confined to hallowed walls, some fit the current narrative.

I caught my first glimpse of ball-striking genius, Moe Norman in the nineteenth hole of the Maple Downs Golf and Country Club in Richmond Hill during the 1964 Ontario Junior Championship. Moe liked to watch kids play. I caddied that day for my brother who eagled the par-five ninth just before the turn. We sped to the clubhouse for a lime Coke®, when we heard a whisper, *"That's Moe Norman over there."* I'd heard the name many times, seen photos in golf publications, but had never seen him live. I glanced to my right and spotted the legend having lunch with a small group. On our way out, Al and I passed within ear-shot of his chatter, *"Money, money, money. 'Gotta play for money … Money, money."* That was the good news. His message rambled through a mouthful of egg-salad sandwich that showered his audience with more than wisdom. It wasn't pretty - but Moe was different, and his status on my list of sports heroes remained untarnished.

Fortunately, we didn't need to travel to Toronto for entertainment. Our nineteenth hole - high atop the Niagara peninsula - provided plenty. One particular episode comes to mind.

Our foursome had just finished putting on the final hole of a sunny day that featured a pleasant breeze and an expanded version of the *Dirty Dozen* – five groups of low-handicap golfers playing for a healthy *pot*. The eighteenth at Lookout Point was an uphill, 321-yard par four. A good tee-shot generally left a short approach to an elevated green cut into the side of a steep hill that led to the clubhouse. The trek to the nineteenth hole was cushioned by a cable-car - present long before my arrival – that was down for repair. It was replaced that day by a pick-up truck fitted with seats, an elevated guardrail on the flatbed, and special racks for bags on both sides. The vehicle rescued a weary foursome every ten minutes, approximately twenty yards to the right of the green. Steve Kozak, in the group behind, settled over his approach as we secured our bags to the truck and mounted the steps that led to the wooden seats. His effort ballooned in the breeze and headed our way. We heard a vigorous, *fore.* I glanced skyward but couldn't pick it up. The ball slammed into the bed of the truck where it rattled among dancing feet and lips. We raised the tailgate, signaled the ascent, and escorted his errant shot up the hill to a table by the bar - still *in play.* Muscles McGurn, as he was known, could have snuffed out all five foursomes with his muscular arms, but he was laughing too hard to muster such effort. *"You guys scattered like a bunch of GD chickens,"* he said in a gruff voice ... and then refused to *play out.*

Some nineteenth-hole antics were more predictable.

I coached golf at Averett College in Danville, Virginia in the early 1970's. The town was famous for its textile industry, Dan River Mills, and local golf legend, Bobby Mitchell, twice a champion on the PGA Tour. When Bobby took a break from competitive golf, he spent the majority of his time in the nineteenth hole at the Glen Oak Country Club, a modest facility on the outskirts of town. I had just joined the club - spent a few afternoons per week playing and practicing – and witnessed the ritual. When Bobby was home, the doors of the clubhouse burst open at mid-afternoon to unleash a mob of Mitchell's boisterous cronies. The bet was on. A dozen golf carts quickly assembled at the first tee to accommodate a single, lawless group. Bobby typically played the best-ball of a large number of low-handicap golfers, and spotted them a shot per nine. When social time was extended, he took them on with a set of left-handed clubs (he played the tour from the right side) ... and won more often than not. The man could play. His talent should have taken him far beyond his one-hole playoff victory over Jack Nicklaus in the Tournament of Champions in 1972, and runner-up finish at The Masters the same year.

Nineteenth-hole antics often reflect the bizarre nature of the game:

- You can do everything right (by the book, by *feel* or opinion) and get a lousy result.
- You can do everything wrong (by the same criteria) and hit a shot that flies true to the target.
- Just when you think you've got it – or haven't - you're wrong.
- Through practice, your ability to identify exactly what went wrong during a bad shot increases, while your ability to identify what went right during a perfect one does not.
- And if that doesn't drive you over a cliff, there's the question of expectations ...

Mike Anderson, an assistant professional at Lookout Point regained his amateur status long before Al and I became junior members. His long reddish-blonde locks and short temper quickly earned him the name, *Fiery* - Canada's version of tour professional, Mark Calcavecchia. One Saturday, *Fiery* was off to a bad start - bogeyed the first hole, three-putted the third, endured a bad break at the fifth and suffered a lousy kick off the side of the green at the sixth. He began to turn up the volume. On the par-five seventh, he missed a short putt for a birdie and mumbled his way up the shaded path to the eighth.

The volcano simmered.

The tee of the signature eighth hole was cut from the side of a steep hill cascading from the right – a hill covered in waist-high fescue and mini-sumac trees. The left side of the tee tumbled steeply to the path from the seventh, its surface burdened by an array of thorn bushes. The former pro selected a four-iron, carefully addressed his ball and shanked it deep into the sumacs. As quickly as it disappeared, he hurled himself over the left edge of the tee to a mix of Tarzan-like screams and profanity. The ball was never found – might still be there. *Fiery* slowly emerged from the briar patch, extracting burrs and thorns for the remainder of the round. The three witnesses to the event (I was fortunate to be one) kept the tale alive in the nineteenth hole for years.

Golfers play their best when they simplify things, and simplification doesn't require lancing yourself over a cliff. When you simplify the skill, mental and physical components of the game, you are well on your way to better golf.

Skill

Skill is simplified by making movement as automatic as possible - free of thought - and the only way to get there is quality practice. Fellow Canadian, Kerry Short was a good player in his youth – shot in the mid-to-low seventies when it mattered – and was ambitious. Tired of finishing in the pack, Kerry began hitting more balls - 200-300 with an eight-iron until he knew *exactly* where it was going ... and then the seven, the six, the five and four iron. The left-hander accelerated through the pack with laser-like iron play that vaulted him to the National amateur scene and a brief career on the Canadian Tour.

In the beginning, as with all players, Kerry went through the process of swinging, adjusting, fine-tuning and perfecting - the skill of golf is a never-ending challenge. My advice to beginners:

- Find a competent professional to teach you the basics of grip, stance, ball position and posture – and return for an occasional tune-up.
- Swing the golf club around what you determine as a *center* (head, chest, back of neck, Adam's apple) that remains at ease, yet *rock steady*, throughout your effort.
- Minimize swing thoughts by focusing on the joy of movement and playing the game.
- At some point in the process, acquire a *feel* for what is - and what is not - correct for you. Hit enough golf balls to trust both the *feel* and your ability to perform when it matters.
- Step to the plate, and pull the trigger.

No one enjoyed the game more than Moe Norman. He was like a kid in a candy store with a club in his hand. His approach, *"Here's the ball, there's the hole, let's play,"* led to the joy of watching every shot sail straight to its destination. Automatic makes golf enjoyable - all you have to do is show up.

Mental Approach

My golf coach at McMaster University excelled in every sport he tried - gymnastics, squash, tennis, and racquetball – every sport but golf. His office was lined with magazines full of tips to satisfy a hungry and desperate mind. One afternoon, Coach and I faced two formidable opponents (both golf-team members) on the elevated thirteenth tee of the Hamilton Golf and Country Club in nearby Ancaster, Ontario - site of numerous Canadian Opens. Coach had the honor. He glanced down the fairway and set his spikes in the turf. The challenge pitted a twenty-four-cleat effort against a tight, tree-lined fairway. In seconds, the verdict was in. Coach hit the worst slice in recorded history - several hundred yards into the woods. Before it landed - if it did - he flipped a second ball from his back pocket onto a tee for a second go. This time, what appeared to be the same swing produced the worst hook in recorded history. The hole, listed at 386 yards - much of it uphill from the fairway – more accurately represented the estimated distance between his efforts. What went through his mind during those back-to-back swings was proof that the mental challenge of golf is as great as that to refine skill.

When you first take up the game, your mind is consumed by fear and doubt: *Can I hit over the water? Can I make this putt to break 100?* Fortunately, confidence improves with skill. I overcame the water-hazard phase by posing a simple question: *"What's the worst thing that could happen?"* The answer was clear: *"I could lose a ten-cent ball,"* and I had a basement full of them. The approach was *fearless*, not reckless - and fearless kept my emotions level.

A client recently asked what I thought about during a backswing. *"My Mother,"* I replied. I am not analytical in my approach – but some are. If you happen to be so inclined, restrict your focus during your effort to *one thought only*. You cannot process more at the speed of the swing.

Physical Preparation

The intent of *Golf Performance Training ... What They Won't Tell You* is not to simplify physical preparation for golf per se, but to identify what produces best results and avoid things that are ineffective. It so happens that the most effective approach is also the most efficient, as follows:

- It directly strengthens muscles that produce movement, the large muscle groups involved in the golf swing.
- It does *not* attempt to strengthen movement patterns (*a futile task*) by emulating the golf swing or its parts, thereby avoiding potential disruption of skill.
- It adheres to the principles of Proper Strength Training – brief, intense, infrequent workouts.

At the same time, it rejects the mythical concepts of *functional* and *sport-specific* training, and those of its offspring, the TPI program:

- That movement can be reinforced by strengthening muscles as they move in a pattern specific to a skill. In other words, that specificity of skill does *not* exist.
- That transfer of skill exists from one movement pattern to another.
- That strengthening small muscle groups is vital to the final product.
- That recruitment of fast-twitch muscle fibers and the production of power are related to speed of movement during exercise.
- That muscle isolation has no place in strength testing, training or in the golf swing.
- That an inferior source of resistance is *adequate* to strengthen muscles to their potential.
- That resistance should not be restricted to a pre-determined path.
- That machine exercise is taboo.
- That intensity of effort (muscle input) during physical exercise should be avoided, or restricted (to not overtax the nervous system).
- That both feet should touch the floor during exercise to mimic the conditions of golf. By observation, parts of the TPI program involve lying on a stretching table. To be consistent (and equally ridiculous), I can't recall lying down during a round of golf.
- That, when possible, you should assume a golf-address posture before, or during, each exercise.
- That improving the performance of *primal* movements will somehow improve the movements of the golf swing.

- That a movement screen is the most effective way to detect functional weakness.
- That improvement in the performance of movement-screen deficiencies through skill training will transfer to improve the movements of the golf swing.
- That the announced results of a movement screen will not invade the head of a golfer in any way but positive.
- That traditional strength training is non-functional, outdated and/ or inferior to a *functional* approach.

What better way to celebrate a day of golf than review the scorecard over a ginger ale.

T, Traditional; *F*, Functional (*using the Stableford system: More points = Better*)

Figure 1: Scorecard

LOOKOUT POINT GOLF & COUNTRY CLUB										
Est. 1922 Architect: Walter J. Travis R.C.G.A. GOVERNS ALL PLAY										
Championship (WHITE MARKERS)					T	F				
HOLE	NAME	YDS	PAR	STK						
1	Skill	423	4	9	**0**	**0**				
2	Strength	135	3	17	**10**	**3**				
3	Flexibility	483	5	5	**8**	**0**				
4	Cardiovascular	447	4	1	**9**	**7**				
5	Body Comp	158	3	15	**9**	**2**				
6	Injury Prevent	405	4	11	**10**	**3**				
7	Balance	526	5	3	**0**	**0**				
8	Agility	175	3	13	**0**	**0**				
9	Abilities	522	5	7	**0**	**0**				
OUT		3274	36		**46**	**15**				

My nineteenth-hole encounters – lunch with Moe Norman, the errant shot of Muscles McGurn, and any wager with Tour champion, Bobby Mitchell - share a theme. If the opportunity presents itself to participate in a golf-performance program with roots in functional or movement training, such as the Titleist Performance Institute curriculum, let common sense prevail - duck.

Proper Strength Training is a better choice.

NOTES

The chapters of *Golf Performance Training ... What They Won't Tell You* are titled with hole numbers, yardage distances, and par standards that represent scorecard values of the Lookout Point Golf and Country Club (now, Lookout Point Country Club) in Fonthill, Ontario during my heyday as a member, from 1963 through 1972.

The photo on the front cover of the book is that of *"The Old Man,"* Walter J. Travis, who won the US Amateur championship in 1900, 1901 and 1903, and the British Amateur in 1904. His passion for the game led to a career as a prominent golf course architect, completing the project at Lookout Point in 1922. I first spotted the photo in the Walter J. Travis room at Lookout Point on a recent visit.

The prominent scorecard in the photo that defines the major divisions of the book – *Front Nine Out, Back Nine In, and A Wee Nip* – is an authentic card from Lookout Point, dated August 29, 1937. The course, then, had a different configuration (6,530 yards from its regular tees) and was played that day by the foursome of Berger, Sands, Watson and a scorekeeper with the initials, AM. The back of the card features a comic-strip golf tip called *Graphic Golf - "a series of interesting, well-illustrated articles that clearly explain how such great golf stars as Lawson Little, Paul Runyon, Walter Hagan and many others handle the problems that confront YOU."* The series was labeled *"...another new sports feature in The Globe and Mail,"* a prominent Toronto newspaper. The card remains in my personal collection and will be donated to the club on its 100th anniversary. The scores remain anonymous.

The scorecard that lies beneath and to the right of the 1937 card (in the same photo) is from mid-1960.

Marlene Stewart Streit, the pride and joy of Lookout Point Country Club and of Canada, was recently awarded an Honorary Membership to the Royal and Ancient Golf Club in St. Andrews, Scotland.

BIBLIOGRAPHY

Academy of Achievement. "Sir Roger Bannister Interview – Academy of Achievement." Last modified November 26, 2013. Accessed June 23, 2015. http://www.achievement.org/autodoc/page/ban0int-1-7

Bannister, Gary. *If You Like Exercise … Chances Are You're Doing It Wrong.* Bloomington, IN: iUniverse, Inc., 2013.

Bannister, Gary. *In Arthur's Shadow.* Carmel, IN: Cork Hill Press, 2005.

Carpenter, David M., and Brian W. Nelson. "Low Back Strengthening for the Prevention and Treatment of Low Back Pain." *Medicine and Science in Sports and Exercise* 31(1): 18-24, 1999.

Chek, Paul. *Movement That Matters.* Vista, CA: C.H.E.K. Institute, 1999.

Darden, Ellington. *Strength Training Principles.* Winter Park, FL: Anna Publishing, 1977.

Darden, Ellington. *The Nautilus Bodybuilding Book.* Chicago, IL: Contemporary Books, 1986.

Darden, Ellington. *The Nautilus Diet.* Boston, MA: Little, Brown and Company, 1987.

Darden, Ellington. *The New High Intensity Training.* New York, NY: Holtzbrinck Publishers, 2004.

De Boer, R.W., G.J. Ettema, B.G. Faessen, H. Krekels, A.P. Hollander, G. De Groot, and G.I. Van Ingen Schenau. "Specific Characteristics of Speed Skating: Implications for Summer Training." *Medicine and Science in Sports and Exercise* 19: 504-510, 1987.

Fisher, James, J. Steele, S. Bruce-Low, and D. Smith. "Evidence-Based Resistance Training Recommendations," *Medicina Sportiva* 15 (3): 147-162, 2011.

Fulton, Michael. "Lower-Back Pain: a New Solution For An Old Problem," MedX Corporation publication, 1988.

Graves, James, D.C. Webb, M.L. Pollock, J. Matkozich, S.H. Leggett, D.M. Carpenter, D.N. Foster, and J. Cirulli. "Pelvic Stabilization During Resistance Training: Its Effect on the Development of Lumbar Extension Strength." *Archives of Physical Medicine and Rehabilitation* 75(2): 210-215, 1994.

Graves, James, M.L. Pollock, D.M. Carpenter, S.H. Leggett, A. Jones, M. MacMillan, and M. Fulton. "Quantitative Assessment of Full Range-of-Motion Isometric Lumbar Extension Strength." *Spine* 15(4): 289-294, 1990.

Herbert, R.D., and M. Gabriel. "Effects of Stretching Before and After Exercise on Muscle Soreness and Risk of Injury: Systematic Review." *British Medical Journal* 325: 468-470, 2002. http://www.ncbi.nlm.nih.gov/pmc/articles/PMC119442/

Hulsey, Caleb, D.T. Soto, A.J. Koch, and J.L. Mayhew. "Comparison of Kettlebell Swings and Treadmill Running at Equivalent Rating of Perceived Exertion Values." *Journal of Strength and Conditioning Research* 26: 1203-1207, 2012.

Ingraham, Paul. "Quite a Stretch." June, 2015. http://www.painscience.com/articles/stretching.php

Johnston, Brian. *System Analysis.* Sudbury, ON: Bodyworx Publishing, 2001.

Jones, Arthur. "My First Half-Century in the Iron Game." *arthurjonesexercise.* http://www.arthurjonesexercise.com./First_Half/61.PDF

Jones, Arthur. "My First Half-Century in the Iron Game." *arthurjonesexercise.* http://www.arthurjonesexercise.com./First_Half/64.PDF

Jones, Arthur. "My First Half Century in the Iron Game." Ironman, December, 1993.

Jones, Arthur. "My First Half Century in the Iron Game." Ironman, March, 1996.

Jones, Arthur. "My First Half Century in the Iron Game." Ironman, May, 1995.

Jones, Arthur. "My First Half Century in the Iron Game." Ironman, November, 1993.

Jones, Arthur. *Nautilus Training Principles, Bulletin No. 2.* Self published, 1971.

Jones, Arthur. "20 Questions: Arthur Jones." Interview by Warren Kalbacker. Playboy, March, 1983.

Jones, Arthur. "Specificity in Strength Training ... The Facts and Fables." *Athletic Journal*, May, 1977.

Jones, Arthur. "The Future of Exercise: 1997 and Beyond." *arthurjonesexercise.* http://www.arthurjonesexercise.com./Future_Exercise/6.PDF

Jones, Arthur. *The Lumbar Spine.* Santa Barbara, CA: Sequoia Communications, 1988.

Jones, Arthur. "The Relationship of Strength to Functional Ability in Sports." In *Total Fitness: The Nautilus Way*, edited by James A. Peterson, 163-167. New York: Leisure Press, 1978.

Jones, Arthur. "The Requirements for Meaningful Testing of Lumbar Function." Risk & Benefits Management. November, 1987.

Lally, David. "New Study Links Stretching with Higher Injury Rates," *Running Research News* 10: 5-6, 1994.

Little, John. *The Max Golf Workout.* New York, NY: Skyhorse Publishing, 2008.

Maglischo, E.W., C.W. Maglischo, D.J. Zier, and T.R. Santos. "The Effects of Sprint-Assisted and Sprint-Resisted Swimming on Stroke Mechanics." *Journal of Swimming Research* 1:27-33, 1985.

Martin, Margaret. "Will the Power Plate Alone Increase Bone Density?" *melioguide.* http://www.melioguide.com/osteoporosis-exercise-equipment/will-the-power-plate-alone-increase-bone-density/

MatthewM. "Walter Travis." *thegolfforum.* http://www.thegolfforum.com/index.php?/topic/5610-walter-travis/

McGill, Stuart, and L.W. Marshall. "Kettlebell Swing, Snatch, and Bottoms-up Carry: Back and Hip Muscle Activation Motion, and Low Back Loads." *Journal of Strength and Conditioning Research* 26(1): 16-27, 2012.

Morrison, R., "Pilates: The Irrefutable Truth." *Synergy.* IART publication, 2007.

Nordlund, M.M., and A. Thorstensson. "Strength Training Effects of Whole-Body Vibration?" *Scandinavian Journal of Medicine and Science in Sports* 17(1): 12-7, 2007.

Ogle, Marguerite. "Core Strength." November, 2014. *pilates.about.* http://www.pilates.about.com/od/pilatesterms/g/CoreStrength.htm

Otto, W.H., J.W. Coburn, L.E. Brown, and B.A. Spiering. "Effects of Weightlifting vs. Kettlebell Training on Vertical Jump, Strength, and Body Composition." *Journal of Strength and Conditioning Research* 26(5): 1199-202, 2012.

Peterson, James A., "Total Conditioning: A Case Study." *Athletic Journal,* September, 1975.

Pollock, Michael, S.H. Leggett, A. Jones, and M. Fulton. "Effect of Resistance Training on Lumbar Extension Strength." *The American Journal of Sports Medicine* 17(5): 624-29, 1989.

Robinson, Louis. "The Psychology of Golf." *North American Review* 165(493): 649-660, 1897. http://ebooklibrary.org/eBooks/

WPLBN0002165094-The-North-American-Review--Volume-0165-Issue-493-December-1897-North-American-review-and-mis-by-University-of-Northern-Iowa.aspx?&Trail=collection&Words=

Rubenstein, Lorne. *Moe & Me.* Toronto, ON: ECW Press, 2012.

Rushall, B.S. "A Summary of Specificity," *Coaching Science Abstracts*, 1992.

Rushall, B.S., and F.S. Pyke. *Training for Sports and Fitness.* Melbourne, Australia: Macmillan of Australia, 1991.

Sage, G.W. *An Introduction to Motor-Behavior: A Neuropsychological Approach.* Philippines: Addison-Wesley, 1971.

Schmidt, Richard A. *Motor Learning and Performance: From Principles to Practice.* IL: Human Kinetics, 1991.

Shrier, Ian. "Stretching Before Exercise Does Not Reduce the Risk of Local Muscle Injury: A Critical Review of the Clinical and Basic Science Literature." *Clinical Journal of Sports Medicine* 9: 221-227, 1999.

Smith, Dave, and Stewart Bruce-Low. "Strength Training Methods and the Work of Arthur Jones." *Journal of the American Society of Exercise Physiologists* 7 (6), 2004.

Szuba, S.F., J.E. Graves, FACSM, K. Hiiemae, and T. Edwards. "Effect of Lumbar Extension Training in Collegiate Rowers." *Medicine and Science in Sports and Exercise* 27(5): S21, 1995.

Tucci, Jacqueline, D.M. Carpenter, M.L. Pollock, J.E. Graves, and S.H. Leggett. "Effect of Reduced Frequency of Training and Detraining on Lumbar Extension Strength." *Spine* 17(12): 1992.

INDEX

1¼-repetitions 178

A

Aaron, Tommy 205
Abdominal muscles 112-14, 118
Abilities 10-11, 15, 17-21, 52, 57, 64, 74,
    76, 97, 163
Advanced training 178
Aerobic exercise 6, 37, 40, 160
Agility 10-11, 57, 63-4, 76-7, 191
Amount of exercise 158-60, 162, 178
Anderson, Bob 197
Anderson, Mike 221
The Athletic Journal xvi, 13, 46, 145
Austin Peay State University xiv
Automatic 12, 208
Automatically variable resistance 137
Averett College xv

B

Balance board 15, 61
Balanced resistance 94, 137, 139
Balsom, Sam xiv
Bannister, Alan xi
Bannister, Sir Roger 181, 216, 229
Barbell xv, 39, 44-5, 79-80, 133-5,
    143, 154
Barre, Paul 129-30
Bartlett High School 129
Bench press 26
Biceps curl 29, 133-4, 150-1, 154, 162
Bodily proportions 4, 6
Body Composition 24, 32, 34, 93, 98,
    144-5
Body fat 27, 32-3, 38, 41, 69, 82, 93, 145

Bodybuilders 46, 48, 158-60, 162,
    168-9
Bodyweight 83, 93, 97, 128, 135,
    159, 168
Bohovich, Reed 138
Bolt, Usain 19
Bone density 191
Bradford, Bill 143
Bradley-Popovich, Dr. Greg 58
Bridgestone Invitational 84
British Amateur xiii, 65, 88
Bruce-Low, Stewart 46, 50
Bulletin #2 161
Burning yourself out 179

C

Calcavecchia, Mark 221
Calf raise 149-51
California State University 188
Calories 38, 41, 72
Caracas, Venezuela xv, 68
Cardiovascular capacity 31, 37, 40-1
Cardiovascular condition 4, 24, 31,
    33, 93, 98, 146
Cardiovascular endurance 10
Centinela Hospital 105
The Challenge of the Lumbar Spine
    111, 120
Charles, Bob 205-6
Chek, Paul 56, 62, 67, 97, 229
Chin-ups 150-1, 161-2
Chronic Disuse Atrophy 103, 120
Chu, Donald 80, 84
Clarkesville, TN xiv, 213
The Colorado Experiment 168

Colorado State University 168

Cooper, Dr. Kenneth 93, 144-5

Coordination 5, 10, 17-21, 57, 64, 76-7, 96

Core 46, 54, 104-5, 107, 112-16, 149, 158

Cross training 192-4

Cunningham, Bill 82

Curls 150, 159, 161

Cybex Eagle back machine 107

Cybex® Dual Axis 91

D

Danville, VA xv, 45, 220

Darden, Ellington 43, 46, 133, 137, 140, 178, 181, 192

Deadlift 151

Deep squat 202

Deficient motor patterns 63

Deland High School 143

Diet 43

Dip 170-1

Direct resistance 137, 139

Dirty Dozen xiv

Dumbbell xv, 187

E

Eagle back machine 105-7

Ectomorphic 164

Eisenhower Trophy 3

Endurance 5, 10-11, 18, 24, 33, 44-5, 47, 83, 110, 120, 157, 191

Erector spinae 118, 150

Explosive training 47, 84

F

False positive 16

Fast 12-13, 44, 47, 49, 79-80, 83-4, 111, 120, 191

Fast speed of movement 79

Fast-twitch muscle fibers 111, 191

Fat loss 168

Faulty movement patterns xvi, 94

Feigner, Eddie 19, 66

Fitness vans 105-6

Flanagan, Jim 71, 79, 81, 84, 109, 112

Fletcher, Pat 205

Flexibility 4-5, 10, 17, 24, 26-30, 33-6, 38, 69, 92, 94, 98, 136, 142, 144-6

Fly 149-51, 162, 192

Forced repetitions 178

Forearm stretch 203

Forearms 30, 132-3, 149

Form 4-5, 12, 20, 29-30, 38, 49, 54, 62, 71, 77, 81, 137-40, 153-4, 156, 166-7

Free weights 5, 63, 70, 86, 97, 136, 138, 160, 168

Full-range exercise 5, 91, 133, 135-7, 139

Fulton, Dr. Michael N. 61, 71, 108

Functional ability 3-6, 8, 55, 96

Functional exercise 62, 69, 73, 90-4, 96-8, 107, 165

Functional training 54, 56-8, 62, 64-5, 67, 69, 72-4, 76, 80, 84-6, 90-3, 96, 98, 104, 146

G

Galaxy 2000 187

Gallager Smith, Jackie 28

Gallway, Timothy 208

General xiii, 6, 10-11, 14-15, 17-18, 48, 50, 52-3, 57, 63-4, 73-4, 120-1, 128-9, 156-8, 162-3

General Brock Open xiii

Genetics 10, 36, 40, 164

Glen Eagle Classic 31

Glen Oak Country Club 220

Glutes 72-3, 106, 158

The Golf Channel 70-1, 86

Golf Digest magazine 8

Golf Performance Training xvi, 15, 88, 98, 143

Graves, James 110, 116, 131
Grip 8, 161, 199-201, 209

H

Haegg, Gunder 179
Hagan, Walter xiii, 182, 227
Hamilton Golf and Country
    Club 223
Hamstrings 27, 58, 106, 110, 149
HealthSouth 105-6
High intensity training 178, 181, 229
Hogan, Ben xiii, 8, 26, 51
Honda Classic 164
Hutchins, Ken 175

I

In Arthur's Shadow 40, 43, 89
Indirect effect 37
Ingraham, Paul 35, 42
Injury prevention 36, 93, 98
Innate 57, 62-3
Inroad 155, 166-7
Intensity xii, 38, 40-1, 45-6, 48-9, 52-
    3, 57, 68, 72-4, 77, 84, 92-4, 144-
    6, 153-5, 160
Internal muscle friction 32, 166, 169
International Association of
    Resistance Trainers (IART) 15
Ironman magazine 46
Isokinetics 85, 167
Isometric rope 138

J

Jarvis, Bob 211
Jimenez, Miguel Angel 197
Johnston, Brian 15, 21, 63, 66-7, 89, 116
Jones, Arthur xii, xvi, 13, 21, 45-6, 50,
    54-5, 66-7, 83-4, 89-93, 111-12,
    118, 128, 131, 165-6
Jump squats 82-3, 85
Jupiter Hills 27, 88

K

Kansas City Chiefs 78
Kaymer, Martin 209
Kettlebell 187-9, 194, 230, 232
The King and his Court 19, 66
Kite, Tom 71
Knudson, George 205, 212
Kozak, Steve xiii

L

Lagunita Country Club 3
Lake Toxaway Country Club 193
LaLanne, Jack 164
Lally, David 36, 43
Landy, John 179
Larrain, Carlos 213
Lateral raise 149-51, 162
Latex bands 70-1, 136
Lavié, Henrique 213
Leg curl 37, 68, 149-50, 152, 162
Leg extension 149-50, 152, 162
Leg press 136, 149-50, 152, 162
Leggett, Scott 111
Leverage 4, 6-7, 135-7
Lewiston, NY 117
Little, John 37, 43
Lookout Point Golf and Country Club
    xi, xiii
Lower back 105, 120, 122
LPGA 28, 33, 105
Lumbar extension 106, 108-12, 116,
    118, 120-1, 123-6, 129, 131, 150
Lunge 151

M

Machine exercises 174
Maple Downs Golf and Country
    Club 219
Martin, Margaret 191, 194
McGill, Stuart 189, 194

McIlroy, Rory 26, 163
McInnis, Gordon Sr. 8
McKenzie, Robin 103
McMaster University xi, xiv, 19, 45, 90, 148
MedX Corporation xi, 61, 116
Mental 12, 53, 210
Mesomorphic 164
Metabolic 5, 24, 35
Miami Dolphins 192
Miss Universe 23
Mitchell, Bobby 220, 226
MLB 77
Momentary muscle failure 5, 145, 153, 155, 169, 193
Momentum 28, 80, 84-5
Mooney, Dr. Vert 125
Morris, Mercury 192
Movement speed 17, 80, 139
Movement That Matters 56, 62, 67
Mr. America 112, 168
Mr. Universe 163
Multi-joint exercise 56, 92-3
Multiple sets 44, 46
Muscle atrophy 83, 109, 121
Muscle balance 112-14
Muscle endurance 24, 33, 44-5, 47, 157
Muscle fatigue tests 122
Muscle fiber-type 120
Muscle growth 92, 167
Muscle isolation 56, 103, 113, 120, 128, 138
Muscle-mass/body-fat ratio 38
Muscle soreness 36, 43, 167
Muscle strength 4, 6-7, 24, 27-8, 33, 40-1, 44-5, 52, 58, 98, 119, 129, 136, 157, 163
Muscles 4-6, 14-15, 28-32, 34-41, 58-9, 70-4, 80-2, 91-4, 103-14, 116-25, 127-9, 133-6, 148-9, 152, 158-60

N

National Academy of Sports Medicine (NASM) 54
National Strength and Conditioning Association (NSCA) 80
Nautilus Lower-Back machine 109, 111, 119, 121, 123, 125
Nautilus Multi-Exercise machine 170-1
Nautilus-only group 144-6
Nautilus Sports/Medical Industries 45, 68, 71, 133, 143, 162
Nautilus Time Machine 45
NBA 82
Neck 62, 79, 144, 148, 198, 205
Negative 16-17, 28, 33, 82, 137, 139, 143, 145, 151, 155, 166-70, 178
Nelson, Byron 51
Nelson, Dr. Brian 128
Neurological efficiency 4, 6
New York Giants 138
New York Times 128
NFL 78-9, 138
Niagara escarpment xiv, 87
Niagara Falls Country Club xv, 117
Niagara peninsula xiii
Nicklaus, Jack 72, 158
Norfolk Golf and Country Club 211
Norman, Moe 7-8, 51, 53-4, 65, 86, 133, 141, 143, 146, 219
Nowak, Dick 129-30
Number of repetitions 5, 47, 145, 156-7, 161

O

Obliques 104, 113, 149-50, 158
Olde Mill Golf Club 98
Orlando, Fl 7, 54, 65
Outright hard work 52
Overhead press 39, 149-51, 161-2

Overhead reach 198
Overload 6, 52-3, 58-9, 91, 95-6
Overtraining 159

P

Palacios, Barbara 23
Parnevik, Jesper 97
Parnevik, Jessica 90
Peak strength 127-8
Pelvic restraint 120, 122
Pelvic Rotation 119, 122-3
Pelvic stabilization 116, 124-5, 131
Peoples, Bob 167
Performance training xvi, 15, 60, 67,
    69, 71, 88, 98, 138, 143
Peterson, James A. 55, 144, 147
PGA xiii, 26, 28, 33, 39, 51, 64, 71, 78,
    90, 105, 117, 141, 163-4
PGA Championship 163
Pilates 27, 54, 72, 116
Pinehurst Country Club 39
Player, Gary xv, 32, 39
Plese, Elliot 168
Porter Cup xv, 117
Positive xv, 13, 15-17, 37, 57, 105, 107,
    137, 139, 163, 167, 169, 174, 210
Positive work 137, 139, 174
Potential benefits of exercise 23, 34,
    91, 93
Power 10, 14, 20, 24, 44, 47, 57, 72, 78,
    80-2, 84-5, 105, 115, 120, 191
Power clean 20
Power Plate 191
Pre-exhaustion routines 176
Pre-stretching 137, 139
Presbyterian Pass 87-8
Primal movement patterns 57, 62
Prime movers 149
Pro-style fitness tools 71, 164
Progression 49, 153, 156

Project Total Conditioning 30, 93,
    144-6
Proper skill training 21
Proper strength training 5-6, 21, 29,
    32, 34, 54, 72, 97, 145-7, 165
Proprioceptive Neuromuscular
    Facilitation 36
Protection from injury 33-4, 139
Pulldown 151
Pulley stations 29, 136
Pullover 45, 149-51, 162
Push/Pull 177
Push-up 140
Pyke, Frank S. 22, 89, 99, 233

Q

Quonset Hut 143

R

Radford, Peter 19
Range of motion 6, 27-8, 36, 38, 49-
    50, 80, 111, 114, 120-1, 124, 126-7,
    129, 133-7, 139-40, 158
Reaction time 17, 19-20, 77
Recovery ability 111, 155
Reinl, Gary 111-12
Repetitions 5, 44-5, 47, 49, 53, 63, 71,
    110-11, 116, 143-5, 153, 155-7, 161,
    169, 178
Resistance 5-6, 15, 29-30, 52-3, 56, 70,
    73-4, 79-82, 84-6, 91-6, 113-14,
    124-5, 133-40, 153-8, 164-8
Reverse wrist curl 150-1, 162
Risk factors 120-1
Robinson, Dr. Louis 208
Rockway Golf Club 132
Rosafort, Tim 86
Rotary form resistance 137, 139
Routines vi, 16, 68, 149, 151, 162
Roy, Alvin 78

The Royal and Ancient Golf Club 65
Royal St. Georges 65
Royal Troon 88
Rubenstein, Lorne 207, 215
Rue, Jim 142
Running 18, 31, 37-8, 43, 68, 71, 83-4, 179
Rushall, Brent S. 22, 89, 99
Rymer, Charlie 205

S

Sale, Digby xi, 45
San Diego Chargers 78
Santee, Wes 179
Schenectady putter 65
Schmidt, Richard A. 17, 21-2, 74
Scorecard 225, 227
Seat belt 107, 154
Seated 68, 118-19, 130, 203
Seated groin stretch 203
Seated hamstring stretch 203
Sellig, Bob 130
Senior Tour 76, 105
Sets xiv, 5, 44, 46, 49, 159, 169, 178, 208
Shankland, Craig 207
Sherk, Cathy xi
Short, Kerry 222
Sifford, Charlie 205
Single-joint exercises 72
Skill xvi, 4-11, 13-21, 23-6, 28, 50-4, 57, 59-65, 68-70, 73-7, 81-2, 90-1, 94-8, 115, 142-3
Skill acquisition 15, 52
Slow 4-5, 12, 47, 49, 76, 79-80, 83, 120, 154, 156, 166, 175, 178
Slow speed of movement 49, 79, 154
Slow-twitch muscle fibers 83, 120
Smaller muscle groups 152
Smith, Dave 46, 50
Snead, Sam 51

Soleus stretch 201
Sommerville, Barry 106
Specificity xvi, 6, 9, 13, 17, 19, 21-2, 52-3, 60, 64, 67, 74-5, 80, 85, 89
Speed 10-11, 26-7, 29-30, 32-3, 47, 49, 62-3, 74, 78-84, 95, 117, 137, 139-40, 153-4, 157
Speed of movement 30, 32, 47, 49, 62-3, 74, 78-84, 86, 137, 153-4, 157
Sport-specific training 13, 54
Squat 56, 59, 69, 149-51, 161, 202
Standing hamstring stretch 201
Stewart Streit, Marlene xi, xiii, 8
Sticking point 135
Stiff-legged deadlift 161
Stranahan, Frank 39
Street, Jeff 28
Strength 3-8, 23-30, 32-41, 44-8, 50-6, 72-5, 89-94, 108-12, 114-19, 121-9, 133-8, 143-50, 155-7, 163-6, 168-9
Strength gains 47, 84, 86, 91-2, 126
Strength maintenance 126-7
Strength potential 25, 60, 72, 157
Strength training principles 48, 140, 150, 152-3, 192
Stretches 37, 197, 202, 204
Stretching xii, xvi, 26-30, 35-8, 42-3, 69-70, 92, 105, 107, 117, 137-9, 163, 197
Super Slow 175
Supplemental exercise 42
Suspension training (TRX) 183
Swiss ball 15, 60, 63, 78, 112, 128, 164
Syracuse University 110, 112

T

Tendons 29-30, 36
Titleist Performance Institute 69
Toledo strongman 39
Traditional exercise 54, 62, 68, 97-8, 104-5

Trainable performance factors 42

Training xvi, 3-10, 13-16, 20-4, 28-34,
        38-41, 45-8, 50-62, 67-86, 88-99,
        103-7, 112-16, 123-7, 140-8, 156-66

Transfer xvi, 11, 13, 15-21, 57, 60, 63-4,
        70, 74-7, 85, 106, 115, 162

Travis, Walter J. xi, xiii

Trevino, Lee 214

Triceps muscle 152

Trowbridge, Ken 7

Truman State University 188

Trunk rotation 200

TRX 72, 136, 139, 185

U

Ultimate Speed 81-2

The United States Military
        Academy 144

Universal machines 5

University of California at San Diego
        104, 118

University of Florida 104-6, 110, 112,
        114, 118, 123, 134, 156

University of Liverpool 46

University of North Carolina at
        Greensboro xi, xv

University of Waterloo 189

Unrestricted speed of movement 137

Upper arms 152, 158

US Amateur xiii, 65

V

Valhalla Golf Club 163

Variable resistance 118, 137, 139

Venezuelan Golf Federation 3, 23

Viator, Casey 112, 168

W

Wakeham, Tim 70

Warm up 35, 117

The Washington Post 120

Water ski 111

Weider, Joe 44

Weighted balls 136

Weslock, Nick 132, 140

West Point, NY 93

White, Joseph III 129-30

William's flexion exercises 103

Woods, Tiger 8, 26, 39, 83-4, 86,
        117, 163

Work xi-xii, 4, 17-19, 26, 45-6, 48, 50,
        54, 61-2, 80-1, 134, 154-5, 158-9,
        166-7, 169

Workout 3, 5, 16, 43, 45, 49, 53, 68-9,
        77, 145, 150-3, 156-8, 160-2, 169

World Team Amateur Championship
        xvi, 3

Wrist curl 150-1, 162

Y

Yoga 27, 54, 72

Z

Z, Steve 110, 112

www.ingramcontent.com/pod-product-compliance
Lightning Source LLC
Chambersburg PA
CBHW030426290526
45786CB00001B/156